HOW TO TALK TO YOUR
CHILD'S DOCTOR

HOW TO TALK TO YOUR
CHILD'S DOCTOR

A Handbook for Parents

CHRISTOPHER M. JOHNSON, MD

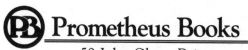
Prometheus Books

59 John Glenn Drive
Amherst, New York 14228–2119

Published 2008 by Prometheus Books

Inquiries should be addressed to
Prometheus Books
59 John Glenn Drive
Amherst, New York 14228–2119
VOICE: 716–691–0133, ext. 210
FAX: 716–691–0137
WWW.PROMETHEUSBOOKS.COM

12 11 10 09 08   5 4 3 2 1

Library of Congress Cataloging-in-Publication Data

How to talk to your child's doctor : a handbook for parents / Christopher M. Johnson.
    p. cm.
    Includes index.
    ISBN 978–1–59102–619–8 (pbk.)
    1. Pediatrics—Popular works. 2. Communication in pediatrics. I. Johnson, Christopher M.

RJ61.H83 2008
618.92—dc22

2008007797

Printed in the United States of America on acid-free paper

CONTENTS

ACKNOWLEDGMENTS

I thank my wife, Jennie, for her constant encouragement to write down all the things I have learned from my small patients and their parents—the result is this book. I thank my agent, Anne Devlin, for her confidence that I could do this, and my editor, Julia DeGraf, for her perceptive and thorough editing job. I also thank the imaging department of St. Cloud Hospital, St. Cloud, Minnesota, for providing the figures of normal X-rays and scans. Finally, I thank the thousands of parents I have met over the years who trusted me to care for their children.

INTRODUCTION

L ike ships passing in the night. This expression can often be used to describe the encounter between the parents of a sick or injured child and the doctor. Parents do their best to describe the child's problem, while the doctor listens and tries to fit what he is hearing into a diagnostic box. Usually, the exchange results in the child getting what is needed, but too often this happens in spite of, rather than because of, the dynamics of the encounter in the examining room. This problem is heightened by a situation in which parents commonly find themselves: because their child does not regularly see the same doctor, the parents often do not know the doctor, and the doctor does not know their child.

There is a common and pernicious communication difficulty between doctors and parents. The problem is not one of language, although medical jargon sometimes interferes with communication; the root of the problem is viewpoint. Few parents understand what we doctors are listening for when we talk to them, how we actually examine their child, and how we combine these findings with laboratory tests to solve their child's medical problem. Likewise, doctors must try to understand how they are coming across to parents.

It is clear to me that a principal cause of failed communication between parents and doctors is that the basis of medical decision making is mysterious to most nonphysicians. However, one does not need the knowledge base of doctors to understand how we use that knowledge in treating a sick child. Any parent can gain the understanding of how the process works. This book will give you that understanding. It will admit you to a doctor's mental universe. It is the result of real-life experiences I have had with parents of sick children about their frustrations in understanding just how doctors think—how we formulate and solve problems. The book will not make a doctor of out of you, but it will make you a better partner in the diagnostic and therapeutic experience when your child is sick, and thereby ensure that your child gets the best care possible. Of course, nothing in this book should be construed as specific advice about your child's particular medical situation. You should always consult a physician for such advice.

Chapter 1

LIKE SHIPS PASSING IN THE NIGHT

Imagine yourself in this scenario. It is the middle of the night and your two-year-old son has just awakened you with his crying. When you go into his room, you find him to be fussy and uncomfortable. You cannot really tell what is bothering him and you are not even sure he recognizes you; his eyes have a glazed look to them. He cannot tell you if anything hurts, but his forehead feels warm to the touch—he has a fever. He also has a rash all over his chest and belly that was not there when you put him to bed. All this comes as a complete surprise to you because he seemed fine six hours ago.

Even though it is the middle of the night, you think he is too sick to wait until morning to call his regular doctor, so you decide to take him to the emergency department at the nearest hospital. It is almost certain that you will meet a doctor there who does not know you or your child at all. Will you be able to talk to this stranger and explain the problem well enough so your child gets the best care?

Or imagine yourself in this scenario. For the past month, your four-year-old daughter has been increasingly tired and listless. Her appetite has decreased, and she has started taking afternoon naps again. When you ask her what is wrong—and you have been worriedly doing that more and more—she does not complain about anything in particular. You know something is wrong, but you have no idea what it could be, so you schedule an appointment with her regular doctor. The doctor is so busy that she has only a brief appointment slot to see your child. Will you be able to make the best use of this short time with the doctor to communicate how concerned you are and why?

These two scenarios represent real-life situations and provide examples of how difficult it can be for parents to deal with doctors in situations other than a regular appointment. The communication problem can cut both ways: a doctor who has never seen your child before will begin her evaluation without the benefit of knowing anything about you or your child.

The first of these two scenarios is straightforward for a doctor. The second, however, may not be; it is potentially a much more complicated problem. It is made doubly challenging for the doctor if she does not know you or your child. Children present unique challenges to physicians. Our little patients can rarely tell us what is bothering them; we rely on observation, seasoned by experience, to figure out the problem. It is a medical cliché that pediatrics is a little like veterinary medicine in the sense that our patients cannot explain their problem. We doctors very much need parents' help to figure out what is wrong, but few parents understand how doctors actually think, how we conceptualize and solve problems. Once again, however, the communication difficulty can be two-sided; doctors may not understand what parents are telling them because we become so accustomed to our own way of thinking.

The issue is not one of language; it is rather one of viewpoint.

Both sides—doctors and parents—often think they understand each other. But like those famous ships that pass each other in the night, communicating only with blinking lights dimly seen through the fog, parents and doctors often do not understand one another. In these days when visits to the doctor are increasingly brief and harried, effective communication between parents and their child's physician is more important than ever.

Misunderstanding between doctors and families is frustrating, wasteful, and sometimes even dangerous. There are various reasons why it can happen, but often the misunderstanding derives from the fact physicians inhabit our own mental world with its own rules and procedures. It is a different world from that of nonphysicians and thus it can be difficult for both physician and nonphysician to communicate.

Practicing medicine is in some ways an art. This is true of some aspects of medicine more than it is of others, but the fact remains: medicine makes use of science, even relies on science, but it is not science. It is a mixture of experience, intuition, common sense, and blind guesswork—all guided by science but not entirely controlled by hard scientific facts. Most parents do not understand this. Films and television shows have done medicine no favors by portraying what we do as highly scientific. At the other extreme, there are movies and shows that depict doctors as bumbling idiots, leading critics of our healthcare system to claim that we have no idea what we are doing. As you will see, the truth lies somewhere between these two extremes.

These problems of mutual incomprehension between doctors and families are compounded by the fact that more and more encounters between sick children and doctors take place in hospital emergency departments and walk-in clinics. These are often encounters between strangers, because the doctor has usually never met the child or the family before.

If the child has been seen previously by another doctor in the same medical system, the new doctor may have access to medical records of past problems. This is becoming more common as computer databases and rapid access to both paper and electronic medical records become more available. Parents should not count on this, however. It is possible, even likely, that all the emergency department or urgent-care clinic physician knows about their child is what they, the parents, can describe during their brief allotment of time with the doctor.

The communication problem is not limited to emergency departments and urgent-care clinics. Although such groups as the American Academy of Pediatrics have vigorously promoted the notion of a "medical home"—a central location where a child's entire history is known and understood—many children bounce from one doctor or clinic to another. Often this is because families' insurance plans change frequently. Confusion can result even if the child remains within the same medical system, as these organizations are getting larger and larger all the time.

The emergency department or after-hours urgent-care clinic is particularly fraught with the potential for miscommunication between a doctor and the parents of a sick child. These are often high-volume places, where there is considerable emphasis on throughput —getting the children seen, treated, and out the door. The interactions can also start out on the wrong foot when a harried doctor meets worried parents who have been waiting, sometimes for hours. Too often both sides are already cranky before the interview even starts. But before we examine the dynamics of how communication between doctors and patients can go awry, it helps first to understand a little bit about how emergency and urgent-care facilities are usually organized.

Once through the emergency department door and registered with a clerk, the first medical person a parent with a sick child meets is a nurse. The waiting children are typically sorted by how sick they appear to the nursing staff. It is not first-come, first-served; the sickest get seen first. This is called *triage*, a term derived from a French word meaning to prioritize patients into thirds based on the urgency of their needs: the critically ill, the seriously ill, and the not-so-ill. This is how it should be.

The triage nurse typically has only a few minutes, sometimes even less than a minute, to spend with the child. The nurse asks the parents a few questions, glances at the child, and makes a quick assessment to see how ill the child looks. Sometimes at this point the nurse checks the child's temperature, pulse rate, and breathing rate; sometimes this happens later. If the child is in one of the top tiers of the triage pyramid, the nurse hustles the child to the examination area. If, like most children, the child is in the least-ill third of the triage pyramid, the family then waits to be seen, sometimes for a very long time.

When the family is called back to the examining room, a nurse again asks the parents a few questions. The child and family then wait some more; since the typical emergency department has many more examining rooms than it has doctors, families wait in one of these rooms until the doctor gets to them. Finally, the doctor comes to the examining room door, looks at the brief note written by the nurse—which usually consists of statements like "fever for three days," "coughing for a week," or "vomiting since yesterday"—and then whisks into the room.

Parents should realize that this doctor they are meeting nearly always has several other things on her mind besides their child. The doctor in a busy emergency department is typically juggling the problems of other children in other rooms at the same time she is evaluating your child. For example, she may also be thinking about a child sent off to the radiology department for X-rays, about another with blood test results pending, and perhaps a third awaiting an evaluation from a surgeon about possible appendicitis. It is difficult for an emergency department doctor to approach your child with a totally clear mind—there are always going to be competing issues. In a very busy emergency department, it is often nearly impossible to have a brief interview with a doctor that is not interrupted by others calling the doctor, who for the moment is *your child's* doctor, away to the telephone or out into the corridor for a discussion.

It is not an ideal system, but it is what we have. It usually works, but it is easy to see how this built-in pressure and chaos can sometimes lead to problems. The best way to understand this situation is through detailed examples of what can happen when both sides think they are hearing each other but are not. These misunderstandings are rarely anyone's fault—everyone wants to give every child the best possible care—but the system can conspire against our good intentions.

The following stories describe real children whose problems for some time defied several doctors' efforts to understand them. In some instances, I have structured parts of the encounters between families and doctors as a dialogue to better illustrate the issue. In all cases, however, I had long conversations with the parents, and the stories occurred pretty much as I have written them. Please note that I have not used the children's real names in any of these examples.

CASE #1: NOT YOUR USUAL CROUP

Johnny was a happy, inquisitive two-year-old who had generally been healthy since birth. He had a few ear infections and a couple of rashes but no previous difficulties of any sort with his breathing. One day he got a typical toddler cold, what physicians call a URI— upper respiratory infection. He had the standard runny nose and cough, in spite of which he was active and playful. After a few days of this, he seemed to his mother to be getting better. However, the next day he suddenly began to cough quite forcefully, so she took him to the emergency department of the hospital on a Sunday evening.

Late in the day on a Sunday is a very busy time for most pediatric emergency departments. Many parents wait out their child's symptoms through the weekend, then come to the doctor just before Monday morning, with its work, school, and day care concerns. I am not condemning parents for doing this; it is a natural thing to do. But it does add to the staff workload when large numbers of children arrive at the same time. Late Sunday afternoon and early evening is such a time.

The triage nurse placed Johnny in the bottom third of the list, so he and his mother took their place in the line to see the doctor. After three hours in the waiting room, they finally made it back to the examining room, where they waited another half hour before the doctor came in, cordial but obviously very busy. Their initial exchange went something like this:

"Hello, I'm Dr. Jones. So Johnny's been coughing for two days?"

"Yes, he started out with—"

"What's the cough like? Dry or thick with mucus?"

As he spoke, the doctor whipped his stethoscope from his neck and listened to Johnny's chest. Since the doctor asked questions while his stethoscope was still in his ears, Johnny's mother was not even sure the doctor could hear her answers.

"Pretty dry."

"Anyone at home sick?"

"His brother has a cold."

"Any fever?"

"I'm not sure. He never felt warm."

"Well, he hasn't got a fever now," said the doctor, as he put his stethoscope away and took a ten-second look in the child's throat and both his ears. "Johnny has croup, a viral infection that makes him cough. We'll give him a breathing treatment and a shot of steroids. If he's better in an hour or so we'll send him home. I'll check back on him later to see how he's doing."

With that, the doctor zipped out of the room. In the hallway he wrote some quick orders for the medicines and told the nurse to give Johnny's mother an informational handout to read about croup while they waited for the medicines to work. Then the doctor moved on to the next patient. The entire encounter probably took only five minutes.

The doctor made such a quick diagnosis based upon several things. It was winter, and he had already seen dozens of children with croup over the past few days. Croup is a common illness, especially during the winter. The doctor thus began moving down his diagnostic decision path toward croup even before he went into the examination room, especially because he could even hear Johnny's typical "croupy" cough, along with a raspy breathing sound called *stridor*, from out in the hallway. In effect, the doctor went into the examination room looking for reasons Johnny did *not* have croup; when his quick evaluation showed none, that was that—the diagnosis was croup.

Johnny's mother told me later that she recalled the doctor was cordial but clearly in a hurry. Body language is important at times like this, and doctors in emergency departments often do not sit down beside the patient. This one did not. Standing over the patient is not conducive to conversation. He asked his questions while examining Johnny, and was not really looking at his mother when he asked them. That, too, does not encourage a parent to volunteer much additional information. Johnny's mother told me later she did not want to bother the doctor with questions—he was so clearly very busy. They had already been waiting a long time, and she was anxious for Johnny to get the breathing treatment, the steroid injection, and then get home.

The doctor was a competent, well-trained physician. From his viewpoint, he was probably relieved by his quick scan of Johnny's chart in the hall and the sound of the child's cough through the door. To him it meant this case would be a quick one, allowing him to move on to sicker children with more challenging problems. What parents should understand is that doctors in this setting are usually making diagnostic decisions in their minds before they even see the patient, and this process continues from the moment they walk in the examination room, even before anybody says anything. As you will read, Johnny's case turned out not to be straightforward at all. Better communication would have helped, particularly if Johnny's mother knew how to present the information in a way that gave important signals to the doctor.

The breathing treatment, a cool mist containing a medicine called epinephrine, made Johnny's breathing better. Croup causes inflammation of the airway just below the vocal cords, and epinephrine shrinks some of the inflamed tissues there, allowing air to flow better in and out of the lungs. He also got an injection of dexamethasone, a steroid medicine that reduces swelling in the airway. The emergency department kept Johnny for another couple of hours to make sure he did not need any more treatments. The doctor then did a fifteen-second repeat examination, found the stridor to be gone, and sent Johnny home.

Johnny's mother agreed that he was significantly better after the breathing treatment and the steroids. Over the next couple of days, however, Johnny never returned to normal. He still had a cough that made him sound like a seal. The cough was worse at night when he lay down, although the odd thing about the cough was that it came and went suddenly at intervals. He still looked well otherwise and had no fever or other symptoms. The runny nose went away completely, but still he had that raspy cough. Johnny's mother made an appointment for the child to see his regular doctor the next day, but that night his cough was as bad as it had been at the beginning. He also was having more breathing troubles—the stridor was back. She decided to take him back to the emergency department.

Their wait in the emergency department was again several hours before Johnny made it back to the examination room. The doctor on duty was a different doctor than had seen the child the first time, although this doctor did at least have a copy of the record of Johnny's first visit. Later I read the note from the previous doctor. It was brief, as they usually are in situations like this: *Typical croup following two days of URI* (upper respiratory infection); *responded to epi neb* (the breathing treatment); *home after IM decadron* (the steroid shot); *follow-up with PCP prn* (to see his regular doctor as needed).

The new emergency department doctor looked at this note, again heard Johnny's cough and stridor from the hallway, and knew what to do even before she went into the examination room. This doctor was even more harried and harassed than the previous one had been—it was a particularly busy night. She ordered another epinephrine breathing treatment for Johnny even before seeing the child and then went on to another child, planning to come back in fifteen minutes or so to see Johnny after the treatment had time to do its work. She also ordered an X-ray of the child's chest and upper airway to make sure there was no pneumonia present, even though she knew this was quite unlikely in the absence of fever.

When the doctor got back to Johnny, he was indeed better; his cough was less harsh and his stridor was once more gone. His X-ray was normal. The doctor decided Johnny's problem was most likely persistent viral croup, being just a longer, more severe case of this common illness. Even though she thought this was the cause of the cough, the doctor hedged her bets by treating Johnny for another possibility—asthma. Asthma generally causes wheezing in the lungs. Sometimes, however, children with asthma manifest their illness with a very prominent cough, but only mild wheezing.

When the doctor sent Johnny home this time it was with a prescription for a five-day treatment course with oral steroids, rather than the single shot he got last time. This would treat both croup and asthma. She also prescribed inhalations of albuterol, a medicine that treats asthma, just in case that was the main problem. The doctor told Johnny's mother to make an appointment to see the child's regular doctor the following week, after the steroids were done, to check up on how he was doing.

Johnny's mother did take him to his regular doctor six days later. She said by then he was again better, in that his stridor had not returned, but he was still not entirely well. He continued to look well, had no fever, and had a good appetite, but he still coughed, especially at night. As before, the episodes of coughing came on abruptly, then disappeared. He also had an increasingly hoarse voice, something that he had not had at first, and which was getting worse in spite of the steroid medicine.

I spoke later with Johnny's regular doctor, and he told me that the one thing that particularly struck him when he heard the entire story was how sudden the original onset of the severe cough was; although the child had a runny nose and a mild cough for a few days, his mother said the cough became abruptly and dramatically worse in the middle of the afternoon before she first took him to the emergency department. Even after a week of symptoms, the cough was still disturbingly sudden in its appearance. The doctor believed this important bit of information meant something was clearly not right in Johnny's upper airway, and that it was time to find out exactly what was going on in there.

Johnny's doctor asked an otorhinolaryngologist—an ear, nose, and throat specialist—to see the child. The specialist agreed that

Johnny's problem sounded like more than simple croup, so later that day he used an instrument with a light on the end to look down into the airway, a procedure termed *bronchoscopy*. It is not a simple procedure, and it is not one entirely without risk, but it was the only direct way to see what was wrong. Bronchoscopy is uncomfortable for the patient and potentially frightening to a small child, so an anesthesiologist first gave Johnny a drug to sedate him.

The specialist found Johnny's airway just below his vocal cords to be a little inflamed, just as one would expect in relatively mild croup. But that was not all he found: beneath one of Johnny's vocal cords and stuck firmly into the side of his *trachea*, his windpipe, was part of the plastic base of a small toy soldier. The object blocked about a third of the diameter of Johnny's airway, and it moved back and forth as the child breathed. The doctor was able to grab and remove the plastic using a tool he passed down through the bronchoscope. When Johnny awoke from the procedure he was already breathing better. By the next morning the swelling the bronchoscopy itself causes was gone, and the child was normal. He went home later that day.

The medical aspects of what happened to Johnny were by then clear to everybody. He did have mild airway inflammation at first, something that often follows several days of viral respiratory illness. But then he inhaled, or *aspirated*, a small piece of plastic that lodged in his airway, and that is what caused most of his symptoms and landed him in the emergency department twice. Because he did really have a bit of croup, and because the plastic probably inflamed his airway tissues a little, the breathing treatment and steroids did actually make him better. However, he never got back to normal in his breathing because his airway was still partially blocked by the piece of plastic. Since plastic does not show up on an X-ray, the doctor did not see it on the image of Johnny's neck taken during his second visit to the emergency department.

The nonmedical aspects of Johnny's case, the social and interpersonal events, are key to understanding why his story unfolded as it did. From them one can easily see what may happen when wellmeaning parents and physicians do not make a communication connection. Johnny's story had a happy ending, but this is not always the case; sometimes communication failures have serious or even life-threatening consequences.

I met Johnny and his mother just after his bronchoscopy, when it was my job to make sure he recovered safely from his anesthetic. I had a chance to talk with her about what had happened. She was not annoyed at the physicians at all; rather, she was mad at herself for not intervening in the situation on behalf of her child, of not knowing best how to communicate with the doctors effectively in the brief amount of time she had to interact with them.

CASE #2: AN UNUSUAL BONK ON THE HEAD

Our next story is about Sean, a sixteen-year-old boy. He was playing basketball one afternoon in the driveway with his brother when he stumbled and fell, hitting his head on the pavement. Sean could not remember anything about the event, although his brother told their parents. Sean did not appear to trip over anything—he just fell down. Sean was a little dazed for a few minutes, but was not obviously "knocked out." Afterward he complained of a headache, so his father brought him to the emergency department. He vomited once in the car during his trip to the hospital.

The triage nurse put Sean in the lowest-risk category because by the time he arrived in the emergency department he felt fine except for the headache. After the usual several-hour wait, Sean saw the doctor, who asked him and his father the routine questions one asks in these situations: what happened, did he remember any of it, what was bothering him now? Sean said he still did not recall the exact moment he fell or even much about what went on for the minutes following, but that he had "tripped over his feet." The doctor examined the boy and did not find anything wrong other than a sore lump on the side of his head. He sent Sean for a special scan of his head (of which you will read more later) to see if he had fractured his skull and to make sure there was no bleeding or swelling of his brain.

Based on his examination, the doctor did not expect to find anything on the scan, but he wanted to be sure. Before he left for the scan, the doctor quickly asked Sean's father a few other standard questions: was the boy "otherwise healthy," did he take any medications regularly, had he ever been in the hospital before, and was everyone else in the family healthy? Sean's father answered that everyone at home was fine and that Sean had "always been healthy." Sean vomited once more on his way to the radiology department, but the scan was normal; his skull and his brain looked fine.

The emergency department doctor made a diagnosis of a concussion, largely on the basis of Sean's brief memory loss. A few episodes of vomiting are also common following a concussion. Very rarely the brain can swell dangerously after an injury like this, and children need to be checked on frequently for the next twelve hours or so to make sure that is not happening. Sometimes this can safely be done at home if there is someone available to watch the child through the night; sometimes such children are admitted to the hospital. It is a judgment call based on the particular circumstances. In this case the doctor admitted Sean to the hospital overnight, to the pediatric "step-down unit," a place where he could be checked on frequently through the night.

I met Sean and his father soon after the child arrived in the unit. He told me he felt better; his headache was nearly gone and he drank some juice without vomiting. As we talked the nurse hooked the boy up to the monitoring system we routinely use in this situation. It measures heart rate, displays the heart's electrical rhythm on a screen, and keeps track of breathing. The heart rhythm tracing did not look entirely normal. It can be difficult to tell much from just the picture on the screen, so I ordered an *electrocardiogram*, a test that tells us what is going on in the heart's electrical system. The electrocardiogram confirmed what I had suspected when I looked at the simple tracing. Sean had a problem called *prolonged QT syndrome*.

This syndrome, which is often an inherited problem, causes an abnormality in the way the heart muscle conducts electrical impulses, and it is those impulses that control how well and how often the heart beats. The heart is a muscle, and it is the zap of electricity that makes a muscle twitch and contract. When the heart muscle contracts it squeezes the blood from the heart.

People with prolonged QT syndrome, on rare occasions, have their hearts simply come to a standstill. The risk of this happening with any individual heart beat is very, very small, but since our hearts beat constantly, the lifetime risk of this happening for a person with prolonged QT is significant. When it happens, sometimes the heart starts up again on its own; sometimes, however, it does not, with catastrophic and potentially lethal consequences. One of the things that increases the risk of the heart stopping is exercise, because exercise normally increases the heart rate and faster heart rates are more dangerous to patients with prolonged QT syndrome.

Once I saw the electrocardiogram, I sat down with Sean and his father to ask them some important questions about Sean's past medical history and that of other members of his family. What they told me strongly suggested that Sean had been troubled by this syndrome for several years. It also explained why he fell and got his concussion.

Sean's father told me that on at least two occasions in the past Sean had collapsed inexplicably. One of these times had been after running a foot race at summer camp. The camp physician evaluated

Sean after the fainting spell, which lasted less than a minute, and decided Sean was likely dehydrated. It was a hot day, the child had been out in the sun for hours, and he had drunk little fluids. The diagnosis made sense; after all, passing out briefly after running a mile in the hot sun is not an uncommon thing to happen to a dehydrated boy.

The other time Sean apparently fainted was a little more ominous. He was swimming in their backyard pool with his family when he suddenly sank below the surface. At first his father thought Sean had just gone down to swim underwater, but after a few seconds he noticed the boy was not swimming. The father fished Sean off the bottom of the pool and by the time they both came up to the surface Sean was wide awake and sputtering. He told his dad he had choked on some water and "lost his breath."

I then asked Sean's father if anyone else in the family had a history of heart problems. In families with prolonged QT syndrome it is especially important to ask if any relatives had ever died suddenly and unexpectedly, particularly at a relatively young age. It turned out an uncle had dropped dead from what was assumed to be heart attack, even though he was only thirty-five at the time and had no prior heart problems.

Prolonged QT syndrome also explained Sean's fall. He had probably experienced what is called an *arrhythmia*, an abnormal electrical impulse in his heart, while playing basketball, and then fallen, striking his head. His two previous fainting spells were most likely episodes of the same thing. Luckily for him, they resolved on their own each time.

The next morning, a cardiologist—an expert on the heart—came to see Sean and confirmed the diagnosis of prolonged QT syndrome. The cardiologist also asked the rest of the family to come in for electrocardiograms, and he identified the same syndrome in Sean's father, even though the man had never fainted before. The syndrome has a usually effective treatment, and Sean and his father both began medication for the problem. This all occurred a decade ago, and as far as I know, both have done fine since.

It was fortunate for Sean and his father that we had put cardiac rhythm leads on the boy, even though we did so for a completely different reason than suspecting a heart problem. This case made all of us go back over Sean's evaluation in the emergency department to see what went wrong. It was clear that communication was the root issue in this situation; there was a misunderstanding between doctor and parent over what each understood key questions to mean.

The doctor had asked Sean's father if the child had always been healthy. This was a general question, phrased in a general way, and most parents naturally take it to mean frequent illnesses like infections, wheezing, and intestinal problems. In fact, Sean had fainted under strange circumstances on two occasions. One might think the doctor should have asked if Sean had ever fainted or collapsed, but remember, the child was there for a head injury, one caused, in the child's own words, by "tripping over his feet." The doctor was already traveling down the simple concussion pathway with his diagnosis.

If Sean had been in the emergency department because he had fainted, the doctor would have asked a whole set of different, specific questions, found out about Sean's previous mysterious fainting spells, and most likely done an electrocardiogram right then. The doctor also would have asked specific questions about fainting and sudden death in other family members. Circumstances conspired against arriving at the correct diagnosis immediately.

CASE #3: A MYSTERIOUS SWELLING

Our final story of the chapter is a little different from the first two. It is not about ships passing in the night but rather about ships that never passed each other at all. It provides an excellent example of showing the importance of good communication between doctor and family. In this case we had no parents at all to talk to for many hours—they lived far away and the child was airlifted to our hospital—so we had little idea about what happened to him before he arrived at our facility. His story represents an extreme instance of what can happen when no communication at all occurs, in this case not because of misunderstanding between doctors and parents, but because there was no communication to be had.

Danny was a four-year-old boy who lived in a remote, rural part of the state. That afternoon his parents had found him unconscious beside his tricycle. They called 911, and Danny was flown by helicopter to our hospital, arriving in early evening. In the emergency department he was confused but conscious. He appeared to have suffered a concussion, like our last patient, Sean. In addition to that, however, Danny had a broken arm. The orthopedic surgeon placed his arm in a splint, and Danny was admitted to our pediatric intensive care unit to recover from his concussion. Over the next several hours, his mental state improved, and it appeared his head injury was a relatively minor one. He also had quite a few superficial scrapes on his skin, mostly his hands, arms, and face, which we attributed to him rolling in the gravel when he fell.

Even though his broken arm was safely in a splint and he had awakened enough from his concussion to drink fluids well, Danny's nurse began to notice a strange thing. His other arm, the unbroken one, was progressively swelling, right down to and including his hand. We had x-rayed that arm, so we knew it was not broken, but we had no explanation for the now rapidly advancing swelling. Then a very astute nurse, one who happened to grow up in the same part of the state as Danny lived, pointed out the swelling looked very much like what happens after a rattlesnake bite. There were no fang marks on Danny's arm or hand, but the large number of scrapes on his skin made it difficult to be sure.

There is a blood test, a clotting test, which is nearly always abnormal following a significant rattlesnake bite; we ordered the test, and it was markedly abnormal. By this time the swelling was worsening so rapidly, we decided it was best to assume he had been bitten. We gave Danny the specific antivenom for rattlesnake bite, and his swelling rapidly resolved. His abnormal blood clotting test also returned to normal. Once the swelling was down, we carefully scrubbed his arm, looking at every scrape carefully. Once we knew what we were looking for, we found buried in the abrasions clear evidence of rattlesnake fangs.

By the next day, Danny's parents had arrived and could help us fill in the details about what probably had happened, although they, like us, first assumed he had fallen, hit his head, and broken his arm. They did not know about the snakebite. Once we told them, though, they were not surprised. Danny himself could not tell us anything; his concussion had apparently wiped out any memory of being bitten, or even of falling.

Danny's parents told us he was an active boy. He was so active that he ranged far up and down the road outside his house on his low-slung tricycle. One of his favorite things was to zoom a quarter mile up the road to a construction site where workers were putting up a new house. His mother always went with him because of his age. She also watched him closely whenever he was outside playing because on a couple of occasions she had caught him peddling furiously up the road by himself to see the action at the site.

Late on the afternoon of his arrival in the PICU, Danny's mother went into his room to get him up after his nap. She found his bed empty and the screen on the ground floor bedroom's casement window off; Danny had escaped on his own. His mother ran toward the building site, very concerned but also very sure where he had gone. She found Danny at the edge of where the construction workers had been digging part of the basement. The child had fallen from his tricycle and was lying on his face, unconscious, with his arm bent crookedly under him. It appeared to his mother that he had lost control of his tricycle and tumbled about ten feet down the embankment that was the partially dug new basement. She called 911 and paramedics flew the child to our hospital.

The parents also told us the construction had apparently gotten into a rattlesnake den, since they saw many more snakes in the area after the digging began. Putting it all together, we surmised that Danny fell from his tricycle, hit his head and got a concussion, broke his arm, and probably landed on or near a rattler, which bit him and then left the scene.

ʓ   ʓ   ʓ

This book will show you how to help the doctor give your child the best possible care, not only by practicing good communication skills but by learning how doctors approach clinical problem-solving, how we use different kinds of information—such as the story of the illness, our physical examination, and laboratory tests—to reach a decision about what is wrong with your child. As you will learn in the next chapter, getting the details of a child's illness is crucial to making the correct diagnosis and providing the right treatment. We cannot count upon having a perceptive nurse around who knows about rattlesnakes.

The key concept for this first chapter is that, in situations such as those of Johnny and Sean, doctors often have already made some preliminary decisions about what is wrong and what they are going to do *even before they have laid eyes on your child*. This is not necessarily a bad thing; after all, the ability to do that is what makes a doctor experienced. Sometimes, though, such prejudging of the situation makes an initial direction down the wrong diagnostic path hard to correct. As a parent, you can help a great deal, but you can best be a full participant in this process if you understand how and why doctors make medical decisions. The rest of this book will give you that understanding.

Chapter 2

THE MEDICAL HISTORY

WHERE IT ALL STARTS

Conversation has been the cornerstone of medical care for over two thousand years. For much of that time, talking and listening to patients was in fact *all* the doctor did; the idea that a physician should actually examine a sick patient is an innovation barely a hundred years old. This notion of talking with but never examining a patient appears ridiculous to us, but actually it is based on a great truth—in most cases, doctors decide what is most likely wrong with a patient and what to do about it based upon nothing more than a conversation with the patient. Of course, this conversation is more important in some cases than in others; after all, a broken leg is still a broken leg, no matter the circumstances of how it happened. The majority of the time, however, that conversation between physician and patient, termed the *medical history*, is where everything starts. If that discussion does not go well, it can disrupt the entire encounter. The examples of Johnny and Sean in the previous chapter demonstrate the potential for this unfortunate result.

In this chapter, you will read about the formal process all doctors are taught to follow when obtaining a medical history. This process is universal among physicians, from the categories used to describe components of the history to the order in which these things are done. The reason for this uniformity of approach is partly tradition—physicians can be quite hidebound in how we venerate traditions—but it also stems from a need for physicians to communicate clearly with one another both orally and through the written medical record. The medical history-taking process is a common descriptive language that has evolved over the years to enable clear communication among physicians.

Even though the medical history-taking process has been developed with physicians in mind, it is extremely useful for parents to understand exactly what makes up a complete medical history interview. Knowledge of the process allows parents to understand what the doctor is asking and why, saving precious interview time from questions the parent would otherwise ask. This chapter will give you insight into that process, which, along with further knowledge you will gain in later chapters, will allow you to be a true partner with your child's doctor.

In the last chapter, the example of Danny—the child who had to be airlifted from a rural area—illustrates the importance of the medical history in figuring out what is wrong with a child and what to do about it when doctors have no history at all. Sometimes this happens because a sick child is found somewhere and brought to the emergency department without parents. Another common, if less extreme example, is when parents pick up a sick child from someone else who has been caring for the child, such as a relative, and know nothing of how the illness began. I have been involved in many situations where this lack of information led to serious problems in caring for the child. The medical history really matters; it affects everything we do.

A key notion about medical history taking is that it truly should be a conversation, with both parties speaking and listening to each other. A skilled physician approaches the history with no assumptions at all about what is wrong with the patient. This can be hard to do in a busy and chaotic emergency department or outpatient clinic, but doctors really must try to do that. You read in the last chapter what can happen when physicians begin the examination with assumptions and conclusions about what is wrong. You will learn in this chapter how to work with your doctor to prevent that from happening to your child.

Doctors, too, must take responsibility in the medical history-taking process. Even though we rely mainly on parents for the medical history, children can often tell us important things, so it is important to listen to the child. I have occasionally been surprised at the answer I get when I ask children what is bothering them, especially when their answer turns out to be quite different from and more useful than their parents' answer.

But before we get down into the actual business of how the doctor takes a medical history, we should consider what can often be a roadblock to the process—medical jargon. Most nonphysicians have encountered this often frustrating phenomenon; nothing derails a conversation faster than the participants speaking different languages, particularly if one participant is unaware it is happening. This can happen when parents do not stop a doctor if they do not understand what he is saying.

Doctors use medical jargon to communicate with one another. To the nonphysician, the argot doctors speak sounds strange indeed. Doctors tend to use fancy words to describe simple things and passive sentence constructions rather than straightforward English. For example, a doctor who says "an operative approach was deemed most appropriate" means "the child needed surgery." There is nothing intrinsically wrong with jargon. After all, most specialized professions have their own specialized languages. The problem comes when a doctor is unable to put aside the jargon she uses to communicate with colleagues when speaking to parents. Parents need to prevent this communication difficulty, since the doctor will not know if you understand or not. If you do not understand, say so. The medical history-taking process gets off on the wrong foot if one participant in the conversation speaks a foreign language and the other keeps quiet about being confused.

There are many terms doctors use that mystify parents. Here is a short list of some of the ones I have found often interfere with doctor–parent communication during history taking. Many parents are loathe to interrupt the doctor, so they let words like these slide by in the conversation without asking what they mean.

> *Distended:* bloated with air or swollen with fluid, as in "His abdomen is distended because of an accumulation of fluid."
>
> *Dyspnea:* short of breath, as in "He was dyspneic after climbing the stairs."
>
> *Emesis:* the act of vomiting, as in "After an hour of being nauseated, she had three episodes of emesis."
>
> *Febrile* and *afebrile:* a fever and no fever, as in "The child was febrile to 102 degrees," or "The child was afebrile; his temperature was normal."
>
> *Hypertension:* high blood pressure, as in "She was hypertensive this morning."
>
> *Iatrogenic:* This is an interesting term. It means physician- or therapy-caused, as in "His rash was iatrogenic, perhaps caused by the medication he was taking for his ear infection."
>
> *Idiopathic:* This is another interesting but common term. It means an illness or injury whose cause is unknown, as in "The swelling was idiopathic; we had no idea what caused it."
>
> *Ischemic:* a body part or organ that has not gotten adequate blood flow, as in "His hand is ischemic from blockage of a major blood vessel."
>
> *-itis:* This is a suffix doctors use to indicate inflammation and often (but not always) infection. Most parents recognize the

common terms *appendicitis* and *tonsillitis*, but the suffix can be added to the term for any organ to show it is inflamed. Thus, for example, we get *nephritis, ophthalmitis, hepatitis,* and *carditis* from the formal names for the kidney, the eye, the liver, and the heart. Doctors sometimes use the term *pneumonitis* for lung inflammation, rather than the more common term *pneumonia.*

Lesion: This is a loose term for any abnormal lump, bump, or spot, as in "The rash consisted of tiny, red lesions on the chest."

Occult: Doctors use this term in a very special way, one distinct from its usual meaning. When a doctor says something is occult, he is not saying it was caused by witchcraft; he is saying it was hidden, as in "The pneumonia was occult—she had no respiratory symptoms."

Organic versus Functional: Doctors often make a distinction between these two labels when referring to a patient's symptoms. By *organic*, a physician means something that has an obvious cause, some clear-cut lesion that explains the symptoms—a broken rib causing chest pain, for example. When a doctor says a symptom is *functional*, she means there is no discernable physical lesion or disease process to explain it. She is not denying the symptom exists; rather, she is saying she can find no physical cause for it. Headache and abdominal pain, for example, are two symptoms that are often functional. It is important for a parent to understand that if their child's doctor says the pain is functional, she is not denying the existence of the pain or that it "is all in the child's head." After all, pain is something everyone's brain perceives a little differently; the same lesion will cause varying degrees of pain depending upon the individual. In that sense pain is always "just in our heads."

Tachycardia: a heart rate that is too fast, as in "His tachycardia is improving; the heart rate is down to eighty."

Tachypnea: breathing too fast, as in "She was tachypnic to fifty breaths per minute."

Terms of anatomical location: Doctors use various standard terms in communicating with each other to describe where something is on the body. We become so accustomed to these terms that we sometimes use them with parents, forgetting they can be confusing.

Superior, cephalad: toward the top of the body, toward the head.
Inferior, caudad: downward, toward the feet (*caudad* comes from the Latin word for "tail").
Lateral: If one draws an imaginary line from the middle of the head down through the middle of the body, this term means away from that line.
Medial: The opposite of lateral, it means toward the imaginary line.
Proximal: near, closer to the center, as in "The proximal blood flow to the upper arm was excellent."
Distal: The opposite of proximal, it means farther away, as in "Although proximal blood flow to the upper arm was excellent, distal flow to the hands was diminished."

ૐ   ૐ   ૐ

The optimal interview between doctor and patient should take quite a while—an hour would be ideal for complicated cases. Most parents know this rarely happens; medical encounters these days are often measured in minutes, particularly if the case is a simple one. The press of time can cause the process of the medical history to be necessarily abbreviated. As any experienced physician knows, however, seemingly simple cases do not always turn out to be so simple. A parent who is informed about how doctors think can help keep us from missing important things, prevent us from mistaking a complicated situation for a straightforward one. The best way to become informed is to understand the medical history-taking process in its entirety.

The first item the doctor writes at the start of the medical history is who is giving it—mother, father, both, child, or someone else. If he is getting some of the information from the child's previous record, he notes that also.

The medical history proper begins with what doctors call the chief complaint, often abbreviated as CC. We do not mean by this that the patient is complaining about anything in the usual sense of the word. The usage is a time-honored one, and as you will discover, doctors do and say many things in certain ways because of tradition. Complaint, to a doctor, does not mean whining; it means the main thing that is bothering the child or that is concerning to the parent. By the time you and your child get in to see the doctor, someone else will already have asked you why you are there, perhaps several times, and will probably have written a brief description of the chief complaint for the doctor to read.

The doctor should still ask you why you are there. Try not to be annoyed about being asked this yet again; there is a good reason to do it. Many parents will think of new things to say, or better ways to say them, during the time between when the nurse first asked the question and the doctor arrives in the room. This is human nature; parents have had some time to think about things once the nurse's questions have jogged their memory, and they often recall things they did not tell the nurse. Many times these additional things constitute key details. Do not be surprised if this happens to you, and certainly do not feel you need to apologize to the doctor for bringing up something you forgot to tell the nurse. It happens all the time.

Doctors are taught to ask about your child's chief compliant in a very open-ended fashion, such as: "What brings you here tonight?" Busy emergency department doctors, unfortunately, are more likely to glance at the nurse's note and say something more direct, like: "So tell me about Johnny's cough." The ideal situation, though, is for the doctor to begin the interview in a neutral, nondirected way, because questions that are too focused in the beginning can easily lead to some of the misadventures you read about in the last chapter. Asking parents what their child's chief complaint is sets the tone for the whole encounter. It is therefore crucial for parents to answer that important question in their own way. An experienced doctor knows this in the abstract, but sometimes in the press of a busy night forgets. No matter how busy the doctor or chaotic the situation, parents need to make sure the doctor hears their own explanation for why they are there.

It is also important, vitally so, to understand what the chief complaint is *not*—it is not a specific diagnosis, because that implies a conclusion. Many parents, and sometimes busy physicians, fall into the trap of describing the chief complaint in these terms. Here is an example of what I mean. Perhaps your child has asthma and has needed frequent visits to the doctor for breathing treatments. On this particular night, he is having breathing problems again, and you take him to the emergency department. You have been through this scenario many times before, and the problem has always been a flare in his asthma. When the nurse, and then the doctor, asks why you are there, you say: "His asthma is acting up again."

That is not the best answer, because it is a conclusion, a diagnosis, not a symptom. Even though you are probably right—it very likely is asthma—the best way to answer the question of "why are you here" is not "asthma"; the best way to answer the question is "difficulty breathing." My point is that the chief complaint is just that—what the patient is complaining about. What hurts? What does not feel right? What is bothering your child?

The chief complaint is a either a symptom, like abdominal pain or difficulty breathing, a physical sign, like a lump on the neck or a rash, or both together, like an itchy rash or a painful lump. In our example, most of the time difficulty breathing in a known asthmatic will turn out to be caused by asthma. But sometimes it will be something else, and it is a mistake to begin the medical history with an assumed conclusion; it is one of the many things that can lead to bad communication between patients and doctors.

Once the doctor is clear on what the chief complaint is (and you should not go on with the interview until you are sure this is the case), the next part of the medical history is called the *history of present illness*, often abbreviated as HPI. It is a detailed discussion of your child's chief complaint. The doctor will often begin by asking a parent some open-ended questions like "tell me about the pain" or "describe the rash for me," but this is the point in the process where the open-ended quality of questioning ends. The doctor has a very controlled agenda, and a parent should not be surprised if she keeps a fairly tight rein on the discussion from this point on. In a sense, the interview moves from the parent-directed chief complaint to the more physician-directed aspects of the rest of the history.

Even though doctors always want to encourage parents to describe their child's particular symptoms in their own words—it is a huge mistake to put our words into parents' mouths—what doctors are searching for in the HPI are explicit answers to specific questions. From the viewpoint of a busy doctor, completely allowing parents to take the conversation wherever they like is a recipe for confusion and annoyance, and it can be a huge waste of everyone's time.

Some parents are naturally better at describing their child's symptoms. Some give answers so brief they convey almost no useful information, whereas others wander all over the conversational landscape. From the doctor's perspective, at least a few parents need to be forced, sometimes seemingly against their will, to answer specific questions and answer them briefly. The natural and understandable wish of parents, who sometimes have been waiting for hours, to tell the doctor everything on their mind can collide with the doctor's need to get key information as efficiently as possible, especially if the setting is a busy clinic or emergency department. I do not mean to excuse doctors who behave rudely, but it is easy to see why a doctor can sometimes appear at least a little abrupt to a parent. Part of the problem is that many parents simply do not know that medical history taking is more than a friendly chat; it is a defined process that must go a certain way if the child is to get appropriate care.

Doctors are taught in medical school the same standard way to zero in on the chief complaint and define it as they take the history of present illness. The details of how to do this vary somewhat with the particular complaint, but the general technique is the same. Using the chief complaint of pain as an example, student doctors are taught to get these items of specific information about the pain from a parent or patient.

- *Location.* Where does it hurt?
- *Radiation.* Does the pain move anywhere or does it stay in one place?
- *Quality.* What does it feel like? For example, is it sharp and stabbing, dull and aching, hot or cold, tingly like pins and needles, or something else entirely?
- *Quantity.* On a scale of one to ten, how bad is it? This arbitrary scale is defined as zero being no pain and ten being the worst pain the patient has ever felt. The doctor often asks the patient to compare the severity with examples of other kinds of pain the patient has experienced before.
- *Duration.* How long has it been since the pain started? Is the pain always there, or does it come and go?
- *Frequency.* If it comes and goes completely, how often? If it is variable, how long does each waxing and waning episode last—seconds, minutes, hours, days?

- *Aggravating factors*. What makes the pain worse?
- *Alleviating factors*. What makes the pain better, if anything?
- *Associated symptoms*. Have you noticed anything else that seems to come and go with the pain?

I have used pain as an example here, but doctors use a similar list of questions to clarify any symptom, from breathing problems to memory lapses. If your child has several symptoms, the doctor will probably use a list like this for each one of them, putting off the decision of whether the symptoms are related to each other until he has considered each symptom. In the beginning, it is unwise to jump to conclusions because at this point the doctor is in an information-gathering mode—conclusions come later.

One of the most important aspects of history taking is the temporality of things, the timing of what followed what and which things occurred at the same time. It is particularly important to work out the relationship between the symptom and potential aggravating or alleviating influences. Expect your child's doctor to ask you to be as precise as you can about defining this aspect of the chief complaint, because it is key in making a diagnosis. After all, for one thing to cause another it must come before it, not after it.

Over the years, I have found this concentration on the sequence of events to be a source of frustration for both parents and doctors. From the parents' perspective, it may seem as if the doctor is overly brusque in getting this information, even to the point of interrupting a parent to ask another question or redirect the conversation. From the doctor's viewpoint, some parents can be frustratingly oblivious to the importance of getting the sequence of things straight, and therefore their rambling description *needs* to be interrupted or their child's problem will never be solved.

This situation is a prime illustration of how misunderstandings can cause communication to misfire. The parents wonder why the doctor will not let them tell the story as they think it should be told; the doctor wonders why the parents will not answer what he believes to be simple, direct questions. Here is an example of what can happen when communication misfires. The specifics have been made up, but variants of this particular conversation between doctors and parents occur many times. In this example, the child's chief complaint was diarrhea and fever. After determining that, the doctor jumps right into the HPI.

"When did the diarrhea start?"

"A few days ago."

"Two days, three days, five days?"

The parent pauses to think. "I think it was last Sunday—maybe Monday."

"How much diarrhea is he having?"

"A lot—all the time."

"Twice a day? Five times a day? Every hour?"

"It depends."

"Depends on what?"

"On how many times I change his diaper. Every time I look, it's there."

"How often is that?"

"Every hour or so."

Having established that the diarrhea is nearly constant, every hour at least for two days, the doctor then moves on to the very important question of the relationship of the fever to the diarrhea.

"When did the fever start, and how high has it been?"

"A few days ago. I'm not sure how high it was—he felt hot."

"Did the fever start before or after the diarrhea?"

"The next day. I remember I had to go out and buy a thermometer."

"How high was the temperature, and has he had fever every day since?"

"It's been at least 101 degrees every day since I started measuring it."

This sort of exchange can start to sound like the famous Abbot and Costello "Who's on First?" skit; the parent answers her interpretation of the question the doctor asked, while the doctor, who has not really gotten a useful answer, searches for various ways to ask the same thing. It can be exasperating for both sides. Neither the parent nor the doctor is trying to be difficult, but parents often do not understand the importance of nailing down the precise facts and order of events in deciding what is wrong with their child, and doctors often are not as effective as they could be in communicating this importance.

The medical history is a conversation, but it is a conversation with rules and a goal. Details matter, especially what happened when, how bad it was, what made it better, and what made it worse. The history of present illness establishes what these details are. The doctor has been thinking in a particular way, often for years; he may not truly appreciate how difficult it can be for a nonphysician to see how important these questions are. The entire exchange can be a situation of well-intentioned parties failing to communicate properly because they do not understand each other's situation.

Once the doctor and the parents have worked out the details of the HPI, the doctor will begin the next step of the process—the *past medical history*, often abbreviated as PMH. Doctors who care for the elderly often confront long narratives in their patient's past history spanning many decades of life. Although some children have similarly complicated past histories, this is rare. Yet even for infants, it is important for the doctor to know what medical issues the child has had because they may play a part in what is wrong now. All parents should know the details of their child's PMH. If necessary, they should write down the details and save them until needed.

Obtaining a child's past history typically begins with birth history, although this becomes less important the older a child gets. Still, a parent of a young child can expect the doctor to at least ask if a child was born early or late, if there were any problems with the delivery, if the child's mother was sick in any way during pregnancy, and what the child's birth weight was.

The doctor will also ask about previous hospitalizations, injuries, or surgeries. An important part of the PMH is finding out if the child has any allergies, particularly reactions to medications. The child's immunization history is occasionally quite important. Certainly if the child has ever had any prior problems similar to the chief complaint for this visit, the doctor will ask detailed questions about that. Sometimes the doctor will apply the same amount of detail to these past problems as for the present illness. In our example of the asthmatic, for instance, the doctor would need to decide what those previous asthma attacks were like and how they compared to the child's current breathing problems.

Parents sometimes get frustrated over what they may see as the doctor dwelling excessively on past issues instead of the current one, but this degree of detail can be quite important in figuring out what is going on with their child. The doctor occasionally must reevaluate conclusions made in the past in light of what is happening now. For example, perhaps what doctors diagnosed as asthma in the past was really something else—a revised conclusion now made possible by the specifics of a child's current symptoms. A good doctor will always be ready to make such a reassessment if needed.

Of course, the main reason for a doctor to spend time asking about a child's past medical history is to consider the possibility of how what happened then might be related to what is happening now. There is another reason for taking time with past history, however, and it is an important one—making sure previously identified health issues really were dealt with appropriately. It is common for a doctor evaluating a child to discover, during a conversation with a parent about the child's current chief complaint, that other, unrelated issues raised in the past were never resolved. Here is an example of what I mean.

A mother has brought her daughter to the emergency department for a cough and a fever that has lasted several days. The doctor soon decides that the child probably has pneumonia—often a quick and easy diagnosis. But as he talks with the mother, he discovers that the girl was diagnosed and treated for several urinary tract infections during the past year. The last doctor to see the child for that problem recommended some tests of the child's urinary tract to make sure there were no abnormalities. This is standard procedure in such a situation. The mother was told to call the child's regular doctor to arrange the scan; she meant to do it, but never got around to it because her daughter recovered so quickly and seemed normal. So besides treating the pneumonia, the emergency department doctor arranges for the needed kidney tests. He would not have known to do that if not for taking a detailed past medical history. Variants of this scenario are frequent.

After the doctor has asked about a child's past medical history, she will move on to what we call the *family history*, often abbreviated as FH. This is a review of the state of health of other members of the child's immediate family. Sometimes it is brief, but other times it is nearly as detailed as the earlier parts of the history. There are two main goals for this part of the interview.

The most straightforward reason is to discover if the child's chief complaint could be related to a condition that occurs in people who are related to one another. Our previous child with asthma is again a good example of this; the condition often runs in families. Allergies are another condition one frequently sees clustering in families. Children get a lot of contagious diseases, often from their brothers and sisters, so if your child has, for example, an impetigo skin infection or a strep throat, the doctor will want to know if anyone else in the family has the same thing. If your family has a complicated medical history, it is a good idea to write this information down so you have it when you need it.

Knowing the family history can be vital for diagnosing what is causing the child's chief complaint. Recall from the last chapter how the family history helped reveal the true reason for the basketball-playing boy's fainting spells. But there is another good reason for the doctor to ask about the health of the rest of the family; a parent's answers may show the doctor a need to address some important medical issues that may have nothing to do with the chief complaint. For example, the doctor may discover that the adolescent boy he is evaluating for a fall down the stairs has two uncles who died of heart attacks when they were less than fifty years old. This bit of information could suggest to the doctor a need to check the boy's blood cholesterol and lipid profile, and as long as he was going to the emergency department for a broken wrist, he would have an excellent opportunity to get these tests done while waiting for an X-ray.

The next item on the doctor's list after the family history is what we call the *social history*, abbreviated SH. It usually begins with a brief snapshot of the child's situation—what grade in school he is in, his favorite activities, how many brothers and sisters he has. The child's environment needs at least a cursory investigation. There are many attributes of how and where a child lives that may have some kind of effect on health, and it is the function of the social history to identify these things. The doctor will also usually ask early in the social history where the child regularly gets medical care.

Consider the child with asthma who is in the emergency department with a chief complaint of difficulty breathing. If that is your child, expect the doctor to ask if anyone in the house smokes or if there are any pets in the house, since both of these things can worsen asthma. If your asthmatic child has been fine for months but suddenly develops severe breathing difficulties, expect the doctor to ask if anything has changed in your child's environment, such as new carpet going down or some renovations around the house. Anticipating these sorts of questions by thinking about your child's environment can make this process easier.

The SH also usually includes information about significant exposures to contagious diseases. The doctor will ask parents where their child spends the day, if any other children in the school or day care center are sick, and if so, with what. This is particularly important information for preschool children, who get frequent viral illnesses because they share toys, cups, and cookies with each other.

Recent travel can be key information. For example, if your child has diarrhea and your family has recently been in Mexico, it is relevant for the doctor to know that. It would also be important to know if your child has been doing things like swimming in farm ponds or if your home has well or city water.

Sometimes the social history touches upon or even directly confronts issues parents may find embarrassing or even anger-provoking. For example, parents may be sensitive about the details of their family relationships, living arrangements, or housing situation. When a doctor asks about these things, she is merely doing a thorough job, genuinely trying to understand the child's illness, and her questions are not (and certainly should not be) asked out of idle or censorious curiosity. Sometimes it is hard for parents to see what the doctor's questions in the SH portion of the interview have to do with the illness, but many childhood medical problems relate in some way to the day-to-day circumstances of the child's life. So a parent should expect at least a few questions of this sort, more if the chief complaint warrants. Doctors, of course, need to do this in a sensitive manner, but it can be key information for the child's care. A particularly sensitive area of the social history is the possibility of abuse and neglect. Emergency department encounters are especially likely to result in tension between doctors and parents who have never met. Many doctors, especially those who do not care for injured children regularly, are themselves often uncomfortable with questions related to this sort of problem, so the tension can be heightened on both sides of the conversational divide.

The issue typically arises with a child who has an injury like a broken bone, especially if the child is very young, and most especially if the child is an infant. All states have very strict laws that *require* a physician to consider (and then report) any *possibility* that a child's injury could have been caused by a caregiver's neglect or actual abuse. In fact, a physician faces severe penalties for not reporting such a possibility. These laws are not confined only to physicians; the reporting obligations also apply to nurses and teachers. The operative word here is *possibility*—the *possibility* of abuse. It is not the physician's job (nor should it be) to determine if a child's injury was nonaccidental. It is the physician's job to care for the child.

What this means for parents of an injured child is that they can expect the physician to ask explicit questions about how their child's injury happened. The very best thing to do is to answer the questions as completely as you can, no matter how angry, embarrassed, or even stupid your answer makes you feel. If you do not know how it happened, say so. All parents have let go of their child's hand when they should not have, or taken their eyes off a child for the split second it took for him to tumble down the stairs. It happens to all of us; no one is a perfect parent, and doctors know that. The two principal things that make doctors wonder if a child's injuries are not accidental are an injury that does not match the history or a history that changes several times in significant ways with each retelling.

The next part of the medical history is a kind of global review of every important issue that might have been left out or over-looked. It is called the *review of systems*, or *systems review*, and is abbreviated ROS. This is meant to tie up any loose ends before the doctor proceeds to the physical examination part of the evaluation. The systems review is a rundown, by body systems, of all the medically relevant issues a child has currently or has ever had. The ROS is meant to be quick, yet comprehensive. Many physicians use a checklist form they can scan, just checking a box on the form if things are normal.

The ROS accomplishes several things. It serves as a brief review of significant issues already covered in the past medical history, allowing the doctor to be certain he has heard the parent's story correctly. It also is a kind of status report on every aspect of the child's body. Finally, it provides a brief description of issues that may not really be medical problems but that still serve as good indicators of overall health. Although the list can apply to any patient, there are a few things in the systems review particular to children. Here is the standard list, along with a few examples of what each category means in terms of children.

- *Constitutional.* This refers to a child's overall sense of well-being. For example, does the child have symptoms like easy fatigue, unexplained fevers, or weight loss?
- *Eyes.* Does the child have any redness, drainage, or vision troubles? Has the child had a vision check or does the child wear glasses?
- *Ears, Nose, and Throat.* Does the child have frequent earaches, drainage from the ears, or runny nose? Has the child had a hearing check?
- *Cardiovascular.* Has the child's color ever looked dusky, or even blue, or has he had any spells of rapid or irregular heartbeats?

- *Respiratory.* Has the child ever been troubled by chronic cough or breathing difficulties? Does the child ever seem unusually short of breath?
- *Gastrointestinal.* Does the child have chronic vomiting, diarrhea, constipation, or abdominal pains? What is the child's usual diet, and are there any food intolerances?
- *Genitourinary.* Is the child toilet-trained? Has there ever been any blood in the child's urine or pain with urination?
- *Musculoskeletal.* Has the child ever had any problems with crooked bones, weak muscles, or painful or swollen joints?
- *Skin.* Does the child have any chronic rashes? Is dry or itchy skin a problem?
- *Endocrine.* Has the child's growth been normal?
- *Hematological.* Any problems with bleeding, such as frequent nosebleeds or easy bruising?
- *Neurological/Developmental.* At what age did the child roll over, walk, begin to talk? If the child has siblings, has the child developed normally in comparison with them?
- *Allergy/Immunological.* Any allergies or frequent infections?

The final step in the medical history is to list the medications the child takes regularly, both those prescribed by a doctor and over-the-counter medicines. It is also common to list the child's allergies and immunization status as separate items at the end of the history because they are so important.

♀   ♀   ♀

You now are familiar with all the components of a complete medical history and how it is taken. If your child is seeing your regular doctor for a complete evaluation, you can expect the interview to cover all of these points. Even if your child is in the emergency department seeing a strange doctor, he should follow this outline, though he may do so in a shorter period of time.

To help you understand each aspect of a typical child's medical history, I've written a summary, just as a doctor would, and using our child with the asthma as the example. If you looked at your child's medical record, which I encourage every curious parent to do, this is the sort of thing you would see, either written out in long-hand (now less common) or as a computer printout of the doctor's dictation (now more common). I have included a bit of medical jargon, although I softened that enough to make it understandable. I also spelled out all the abbreviations doctors would use in this situation. This is a simple case, so the record is brief. Children with more complicated stories often have medical histories that run to several pages or more. Yet as you read this simple case, you can see the logical progression of what goes through the doctor's mind during the interview.

Informant: Mother.

CC: Trouble breathing.

HPI: Eight-year-old male with onset twelve hours ago of tachpnea and wheezing. Mom gave albuterol [an asthma medication] inhaler with some improvement. Worsened again an hour later, albuterol repeated several times with no improvement. Onset four hours ago of chest retractions and increased work of breathing, progressively worse. Onset two hours ago of dusky lips. Brought to emergency department via family car. Received total of six albuterol treatments before arrival. No other therapies.

PMH: Diagnosed with asthma at age five when he presented to emergency department with severe respiratory distress. Required admission and four days in hospital to resolve. On chronic albuterol and fluticasone [another asthma medicine] since. Has had several courses of oral steroids [more asthma medicines] but none in past three months. Has required three visits to the emergency department for wheezing since first diagnosis of asthma but resolved with albuterol and oral steroids without requiring admission.

Birth history: normal product of term pregnancy, birth weight seven pounds. Perinatal course unremarkable. Significant medical problems other than asthma limited to chronic ear infections (four to six per year), treated with pressure-equalization tubes after failing medical suppressive therapy. No ear problems since.

Previous hospitalizations: croup at age two, vomiting and dehydration age three, asthma as above.

Previous surgeries: ear tubes at eighteen months.

FH: Father has lifelong asthma requiring occasional albuterol. Ten-year-old brother has chronic eczema, no asthma. No other FH of breathing or allergic problems.

SH: Child is third-grader. Lives with both parents and sibling noted above in single-family home. Mother smokes but not indoors. Had a cat until six months ago. No recent travel. Multiple children at school have viral respiratory infections. Regular physician is Doctor Smith.

ROS: Other than the problems noted above, ROS is negative or noncontributory except for respiratory system. Besides items above, has frequent, nonproductive cough even when not wheezing, worse at night. Also coughs with exercise. Note normal hearing screen three years ago.

Allergies: Dust, mold, cats. No drug allergies.

Medications:

1. Albuterol inhaler two puffs every four hours as needed.
2. Fluticasone two puffs twice each day.
3. Multivitamin daily.

Immunizations: up-to-date for age.

ʯ   ʯ   ʯ

Now that you know the components of the medical history—the reasons doctors ask the questions we ask—I will make you a fly on the wall for an encounter between a mother and a doctor in the outpatient clinic. The child, a toddler, is too young to participate.

What follows is a made-up dialogue involving real people whose names have been changed. It is a conversation stitched together from many actual encounters I have taken part in over the years. There are misunderstandings and miscommunications here as both sides struggle to understand each other. I will point out where these communication mishaps occurred, but as you read, try to identify yourself where they are and how the participants might have done better. The doctor begins the conversation with the mother of a five-year-old girl.

"What brings you and Sarah here tonight?"

"She just isn't herself. I don't think she feels well."

"What makes you think that?"

"My mother thinks so."

"What does her grandmother think is wrong?"

"She's not sure. I've been out of town for a while and Sarah's been staying with my mother. When I picked Sarah up this afternoon from her house she told me to take her to the doctor."

"What did your mother tell you about Sarah's problem?"

"Nothing more than that—just that she didn't look right and to take her to the doctor."

The interview has now been going on for several minutes, and it is not clear what the chief complaint is. For one thing, both the child's grandmother and mother appear to be under the common misconception that doctors make a diagnosis based upon tests and a physical examination of the child. As you know now, the medical history is the crucial first part of a child's evaluation, so Sarah's mother made the mistake of not getting the story from her own mother. It would have been even better to have the grandmother come with them to the emergency department.

Struggling to identify at least the chief complaint, the doctor collects his wits, probably sneaks a peek at his watch, and plunges ahead.

"Your mother must have told you something about what she was concerned about. Did she say anything about it? Any aches or pains anywhere, any fever, breathing troubles, vomiting, diarrhea, rash?"

"She said she just sat around for the past day and didn't want to do anything. She wouldn't eat much, either."

"Did she have any of those other things I mentioned?"

"My mom didn't say she did."

The two have finally arrived at something approaching a chief complaint, which might be termed lethargy and decreased appetite, apparently in the absence of other symptoms, although we are not sure about that because the child's mother did not ask the grandmother for details. That is pretty vague for a useful chief complaint, but sometimes chief complaints are vague no matter how precise we try to be. To get even this much information the doctor used a standard technique for vague historians: he suggested specific symptoms and asked the mother to respond to them, yes or no. The doctor next turns to his ace-in-the-hole—the child herself. He observes that the child prefers to lie on the stretcher, rather than sit on the chair beside her mother.

"Sarah, do you hurt anywhere?"

"In my tummy."

"Where in your tummy?" The doctor then takes the child's hand. "Can you take your pointer finger and point to the spot where it hurts?"

Getting a child to point to and touch the painful spot is a standard technique to help localize a symptom. It is much more useful than settling for vague statements like "my belly" or "my chest." Some histories are so vague that occasionally, as a last resort, doctors mix the history together with the physical examination and ask their questions as they move from one relevant body part to another. In this case, the child pointed to the area around her navel, termed the *periumbilical region.*

"Sarah, did you throw up today?"

"Five times," comes the answer, accompanied by five spread fingers on an outstretched hand.

With the child's help, the doctor and the mother have at last uncovered a useful chief complaint: abdominal pain with vomiting and decreased appetite. The doctor now realizes he is probably not going to get much more helpful information, especially not crucial details, from the child or her mother. He moves to the obvious solution, asking the mother if the grandmother is home; he then calls her and gets the key details the child's mother should have already gotten. When he hangs up the phone, the doctor knows Sarah has had fever for a day, has eaten next to nothing for twelve hours, has vomited multiple times, and has been increasingly listless. The medical history is key to figuring out what is wrong. Now he knows how to proceed.

As it happens, this particular scenario is a typical one for early appendicitis. When the doctor examines a child like Sarah, he might find the pain in the area where she pointed but also in the lower right part of her abdomen, and that she has fever. He would likely order some X-rays and blood tests. Worsening pain in the right lower part of the abdomen, with fever, an abnormal blood count, and especially some abnormal X-ray scans, would soon land Sarah in the operating room for an appendectomy. Not surprisingly, acute appendicitis is a particularly difficult diagnosis to make in toddlers because children that young cannot tell you much about their symptoms; about a third of them actually experience rupture of their appendix before the true diagnosis is clear.

Understand that I am not criticizing parents such as the hypothetical mother for their inability to give a good medical history. I have met many, many diligent and attentive parents over the years who simply do not know that details like those in the list earlier in the chapter are the what, when, where, and why of medical detective work. Without these facts, doctors, like any other detectives, are often unable to solve the case. The very best way for parents to get their child appropriate and expeditious medical care is to approach these problems as a doctor does, to think as a doctor thinks.

Here is a final example of a typical medical situation we see involving small children. Imagine you have only five minutes or so to explain your child's problem to the doctor, and imagine further you have never met this doctor before. Read the following synopsis of the child's story, and consider how you would present it to the doctor in the best way to conserve precious time and avoid the conversational merry-go-round that was Sarah's evaluation.

Your toddler has been back and forth to the doctor for what seems like weeks. He has had fevers off and on, been treated for ear infections, been given some antibiotics, had a rash, had a day or two when he seemed better only to get worse again. In the middle of this time was a day of vomiting and a couple of days of diarrhea. When he had yet another fever this afternoon, you bring him to the emergency department. You are fed up with all this and want the answer: *what is wrong with your child?*

Before the doctor (who has never seen your child) can diagnose and treat your child, she must first answer one question: is this all one illness, or are these several separate problems strung together? She will use the history you provide, and only that, to determine the answer to this important question. As a parent, you have most likely assumed that this is all one thing, or a series of related things, which has thus far eluded diagnosis and therefore has not been treated correctly. That may be the case, but often it is not.

This particular example represents a fairly common scenario in pediatric illness. Toddlers who have one ear infection typically go on to have more of them, often several each year, especially if other family members had the same problem when they were toddlers.

The problem gets better as children grow and is nearly gone by elementary school age in most children. This is because a child's skull grows bigger and the connection between the middle ear and the nasal passages, the *eustachian tube*, gets longer and it becomes more difficult for the bacteria normally living in the back of the nose to crawl up the tube and infect the ear. The most common initial event is a viral cold, followed a day or two later by the bacterial ear infection. Whereas antibiotics do not help the first condition, they are often prescribed for the second one (although debate over their usefulness continues).

What happened to this child was typical. First he got a cold, then he got an ear infection with fever. His mother brought him to the doctor, who prescribed an antibiotic commonly used to treat ear infections. This antibiotic did not agree with the child's system, and he got a rash from it, then gastrointestinal upset with vomiting and diarrhea. Although the antibiotic caused this distress, it unfortunately did not do its primary job; the ear infection continued to smolder, and the child had renewed fever. So in this case, everything really was all one chain of linked events. The doctor in the emergency department would likely figure that out within a few minutes if you were able to present a clear, coherent history. If you give an incomplete history, as Sarah's mother did, the doctor might never get it all straight and the process of diagnosis would take much longer.

You should use your time before you see the doctor to map out exactly what symptoms occurred when, what was done when, and if what was done seemed to help. Think of pertinent points in your child's past medical, family, and social histories that will help the doctor put everything together. I personally am thankful when I interview a parent who understands this principle and has taken the time to get out a piece of paper and reconstruct the history in advance of our conversation. I like it even better when they talk to me using their paper as a guide, and I like it best of all when they let me borrow their paper afterward while I record my own note in the medical record.

I trust this chapter has convinced you of how important the medical history is for receiving prompt and appropriate care for your sick child. In many ways parents are positioned to be better medical history takers than physicians because parents know their children far better than the doctors do. Parents have not been trained in history taking, but they are usually keen observers of their children. If you can learn these history-taking skills, the result will be better medical care for your child, because neither you nor your child's doctor will waste precious time trying to figure out what each of you are saying and why.

Now that we have discussed the medical history, it is time for the next stage of a sick child's evaluation—the physical examination.

COMMUNICATION CHECKLIST FOR PARENTS

1. Before you see the doctor, try to state to yourself in one or two sentences just why you are there. Use symptom descriptions, not disease categories.
2. Write down the sequence of events of your child's illness. Be as specific as you can about times and dates.
3. For each symptom, write down its quality, quantity, its associations with anything, if anything made it better, and if anything made it worse.
4. Review in your mind the important points of your child's past medical history, particularly past hospital admissions, surgical procedures, and injuries.
5. Write down any medications your child is taking—what they are, how often, and the dose.

Chapter 3

LOOKING AND TOUCHING

HOW AND WHY THE DOCTOR EXAMINES YOUR CHILD

Medical diagnosis is a three-pronged quest for data about what is wrong with a patient. The last chapter was about the first leg of this triad—the medical history. This chapter concerns the second—the physical examination. (You will read about the third leg, diagnostic tests, in the next chapter.) As with the history, the principal reason for parents to learn how doctors examine children is to help them communicate more effectively with their child's doctor: the entire process goes much more smoothly when parents know what is going on.

Considering the timescale of Western medical practice, which began in the time of Hippocrates in ancient Greece well over two thousand years ago, the physical examination doctors do today is a fairly new procedure. It was not until the middle of the 1800s, two millennia after Hippocrates, that physicians began to get systematic about how they examined patients, or indeed even examined them at all. Even in the late nineteenth century, Victorian mores prevented much viewing of another's unclothed body. For most of medical history, physicians decided virtually everything based only on what patients told them.

Surgeons trace their heritage back to practical artisans doing practical work. Being pragmatists, they have always relied on being able to look at the body part on which they were about to work, such as an easily exposed arm or leg. In contrast, physicians were taught using ancient texts and theories; for such classically trained physicians, diagnosis was a cerebral activity, not a physical one.

This began to change when discoveries in physiology—the science of how the body works—made medicine more scientific and when new tools, such as the stethoscope, gave physicians the means to better understand what was going on inside the body. The result was a uniform, systematic way of examining the body, an exercise that has been taught to medical students in a ritual essentially unchanged for the last century. This process has remained unchanged for so long because its usefulness has stood the test of time.

Although performing a complete physical examination requires an understanding of what the examiner is looking for, that is, it requires a knowledge of disease, any parent can learn very helpful things about the process from watching it in action and even practicing it a little. This chapter will give you the insight to do this, and, as with the medical history, it will make you a better partner in your child's healthcare. As I take you through the components of the examination, I will describe why doctors do things a certain way and what common abnormalities they are looking for as they examine particular parts of a child's body. Understanding the how and why of the physical examination will help you to ask pertinent questions during the examination.

The fundamental principle to a good physical examination is to make it a systematic process, performing the exam the same way every time. This is why medical students are drilled over and over to do the same thing in the same order, no matter the patient's chief complaint. The idea is that once the process is hardwired into one's brain, it is more difficult to forget a step in the process. Most physicians who have practiced medicine for several decades feel quite odd when they must, for one reason or another, examine a patient in a different way than is customary. For example, like most right-handed doctors, I simply cannot adequately examine a child lying on his back unless I am standing on the child's right side, as I and all my peers were taught to do. I could train myself to do it from the other side, but consistency is everything, and I would not really trust what I was feeling from the "wrong" side.

This seemingly rigid protocol may strike parents as odd when they watch a doctor examine their child. Certainly a parent whose child has an obvious problem, like a broken leg, will see the doctor go right to that part of the child's body. Even though doctors strive to do their examinations the same way every time, it is also true that we modify a particular evaluation based upon the all-important medical history. This is only sensible. So you will see us pay particular attention to any parts of your child's body that the history you gave us suggests could be key to your child's problem. After that, though, the doctor will invariably go back to the routine and complete the examination in the usual order.

Most of us just cannot perform the physical exam any other way than the way we were taught, and that consistency is a good thing for your child; it makes us less likely to miss anything important. Like every experienced doctor, I can remember times when some obvious physical examination finding grabbed my attention, diverting it from something else that, although less obvious, still needed my careful evaluation. The best way to guard against that from happening is to be doggedly consistent in one's examination technique.

Medicine does have a countertradition to that of using only the history to decide what is wrong with a patient—that is, using only the physical examination to make a diagnosis. This is the technique made famous in the Sherlock Holmes stories. The fictional Holmes had the ability simply to look at a person and determine their personality, their trade, where they lived, where they had been, and much else besides. In fact, Arthur Conan Doyle, the author of the Holmes stories, was himself a physician who said he modeled that aspect of Holmes's character on one of Doyle's own teachers in medical school, Joseph Bell. Doctor Bell was famous for his deductions regarding what was wrong with a patient gleaned only from observing them closely. Sometimes we doctors are indeed forced to play the detective, as you found with the story in chapter 1 about the boy bitten by the snake, but we very much prefer to have *both* an adequate medical history and a physical examination.

Patients, and the parents of pediatric patients, *expect* us to do an examination and rightfully feel shortchanged when we do not do a thorough one. Even if the problem that brings a child to the doctor really is one of those rare complaints that can be completely diagnosed and managed without an examination, parents appropriately expect some kind of exam. A teacher of mine many years ago told me a fascinating and enlightening story that illustrates this principle in action.

My teacher's father was himself a physician, Alfred Adson, one of the founders of the specialty of neurosurgery. The senior Adson was once evaluating a patient who had traveled from far away to have surgery performed by the famous neurosurgeon. The man had a brain tumor, one obvious enough that even the relatively primitive X-ray techniques of the day could easily identify both the tumor and what needed to be done about it, which was to remove it. Doctor Adson left the room after he had finished speaking with the patient to arrange a time for the surgery. A few minutes later, however, his assistant came out of the patient's room with the news that the man did not wish one of the most famous brain surgeons in the world to do the surgery; he would rather go elsewhere. When Adson asked why, the assistant answered: "You didn't examine his head."

The point, as Doctor Adson's also distinguished surgeon-son told me, was that the man expected an examination, even though it would be a pointless thing for the busy neurosurgeon to do; the man needed the tumor removed—case closed. But it was the examination, the literal laying of the doctor's hands upon his head, that mattered most to this patient, not the renowned skill of the surgeon. He did not want to place his life in the hands of a doctor who had not done that for him.

Logically, the physical examination typically starts at the head and proceeds down from there. For each part of the body, the traditional examination comprises several distinct components: inspection (simply looking at the body part), palpation (the actual laying on of hands, plus the poking and prodding), percussion (a special kind of tapping with the fingers that is almost obsolete these days), and auscultation (listening with a stethoscope, if appropriate). A traditional admonition to physicians doing a physical examination is to refine these simple acts: *don't just look, but see; don't just touch, but feel; don't just listen, but hear.*

What follows is the usual list of body parts and body systems that make up the physical examination, listed in the order the doctor performs the examination. I include the whole list because everything on it is important. However, we do find some items on the list are more relevant to common children's disorders than others. As we work our way down the list, I will describe those things most important for evaluating sick children. The categories are:

- Vital signs
- Global assessment
- Head
- Eyes
- Ears, nose, and throat
- Neck

- Chest and lungs
- Heart and blood vessels
- Abdomen
- Genitalia
- Extremities, joints, and musculoskeletal system
- Skin
- Nervous system

VITAL SIGNS

The physical examination always begins with checking the child's vital signs—temperature, heart rate, breathing rate, usually blood pressure, and sometimes blood oxygen saturation. Usually the nurse has already performed these simple tests and written the results on the chart near the chief complaint, but if the results are abnormal, the doctor may recheck them.

There are several ways to measure a child's temperature. The days of the old glass thermometer, which took several minutes to give an accurate reading, are thankfully long gone. Instruments these days are electronic and give an answer in seconds. Oral temperatures are inconsistent and difficult to get from uncooperative children, so we commonly use either rectal temperature for infants or the temperature inside the ear for older children. Doctors define fever as greater than 100.4 degrees Fahrenheit (38.0 degrees centigrade).

Heart rate, or pulse, can be felt over the artery on the thumb side of the wrist in older children or heard directly through a stethoscope placed over the heart in smaller children. Generally, we count the beats in fifteen seconds and multiply them by four to get beats per minute. Normal heart rate varies with age, falling from 120 to 140 in infancy to an adult value of 60 to 80. Blood pressure has two components: the pressure at full squeeze of the heart muscle, or *sys-*

tolic pressure; and the pressure between beats, or *diastolic* pressure. Both are measured with a special cuff wrapped around a child's arm or leg. Blood pressure rises steadily with age from about 90 systolic and 50 diastolic for a baby to normal adult values of 120 systolic and 80 diastolic.

It is important to measure heart rate and blood pressure when the child is calm, since agitation raises both significantly, particularly heart rate—rates of 200 are not uncommon in a crying baby. Fever also normally raises the heart rate, although not the blood pressure.

Respiratory rate, the number of breaths a child takes per minute, is normally about thirty in infants, twenty in older children, and about sixteen in adolescents. Doctors usually measure it like heart rate, counting breaths in fifteen seconds and then multiplying by four.

Oxygen saturation is a measure of how much oxygen is in the bloodstream. It is important to measure this if a child has any complaint related to breathing. The measurement is done using a machine called a *pulse oximeter*, and if your child has any respiratory symptoms, expect the nurse to check this. The oximeter works by means of a small plastic probe device wrapped around your child's finger or toe. The probe, which is entirely painless, emits a bright red light that shines through the tissue and detects how much oxygen your child's red blood cells are carrying. It does this by measuring the degree to which the oxygen-carrying material in the red blood cells is loaded, or saturated, with oxygen.

A normal reading is typically 95 percent saturated or above, although anything above 90 percent is frequently acceptable. Numbers less than 90 percent usually indicate a need for the child to receive oxygen therapy. Values less than 80 percent usually make the child appear dusky-colored or even obviously blue, particularly in the lips and nail beds.

GLOBAL ASSESSMENT

After the vital signs comes what we call the global assessment or general appearance. It is here that the skill of an experienced pediatric examiner is most apparent. The phrase *global assessment* refers to the doctor's innate sense of whether the child is generally well-looking, not so well-looking, or sick-looking. Recognizing the degree of seriousness of a child's illness takes experience and often a kind of sixth sense. It is a crucial part of pediatric practice, particularly when dealing with babies.

It is so crucial that a large amount of research has been done trying to identify a test or other objective measure that can reliably distinguish the very sick from the not-so-sick infant. The results have been disappointing to scientists but paradoxically reassuring to those who still see medicine as an art. The research has shown time and again that there is no measure that can consistently identify how sick a child is, especially a small infant; but rather that the very best measurement of the seriousness of a situation is for an experienced examiner to say: "This child looks sick." Thus the lowest-tech tool doctors have is the most reliable for answering that particularly important and sometimes lifesaving question.

HEAD

When a doctor inspects a child's head, particularly a young child's or infant's head, he first looks at its shape. Some children have unusually shaped heads. Most of the time, whatever shape the head assumes is normal for that particular child, but occasionally this is not the case. More important, especially for a baby, is the size of the head, which should be proportional to the rest of the body. By size we mean circumference, which we measure around the largest diameter of the skull by wrapping a tape measure around the head from the brow to the most protuberant part of the head in the back. We then use a chart of normal values to see if the head is too large or too small for the child's age. The raw number is not as important as a comparison of the child's head circumference with the child's length and weight—all should match. We have standardized charts to determine this.

In small children and infants we also palpate the head, feel the skull, as Doctor Adson's patient wanted him to do. Feeling an infant's head gives important information. The doctor feels the soft spot, called the *fontanel*, to determine if it is too big, too small, sunken, or bulging. A sunken fontanel often means a child is dehydrated; a bulging fontanel can mean excess pressure inside the skull, which in turn can come from some blockage of fluid flow inside the brain or from infections.

The skull bones of an infant are not fused solidly together even away from the fontanel. Sometimes parents notice that the skull bones overlap on their infant's head, forming a ridge. Odd as it may feel to a concerned parent, this ridge is virtually never an important finding, and the bones will move to their normal positions as the child's head grows.

EYES

We assess several things when we examine a child's eyes. We check to see if they look straight ahead or if one eye wanders to the outside or the inside. Such "lazy eyes" often need evaluation by an eye specialist. We look to see if they are swollen, red, or if there is any drainage from them, since those are all signs of irritation and sometimes infection. We check the pupils to see if they are the same size and if they constrict normally to a light shone into them; this checks the nerves going from the brain to the eyes. If possible, we try to get some idea of the child's vision, although this is often not possible in small, uncooperative children. Sometimes it is important to get the child to move the eyes in all directions to test the nerves that control that function.

Doctors use an instrument called an *ophthalmoscope* to look inside the eye. It uses a pinhole of bright light shone through the pupil and then observed through a magnifying lens, allowing us to focus the beam at various places inside the eye. An adequate ophthalmoscopic examination requires two things: a cooperative patient and a wide-open pupil, which is why such an exam can be difficult with an uncooperative small child. Among the things we are looking for are abnormalities of the *retina*, the membrane at the back of the eyeball that collects the information about what we look at and transmits it back to the brain, which is how we see. Potential abnormalities include spots of bleeding or abnormal pigment. We are also looking for abnormalities of the eye's chief nerve, the optic nerve. The optic nerve connects directly to the brain; looking at it can sometimes tell us what is going on within the brain, especially if there is increased pressure in the skull.

All physicians who care for children are reasonably proficient in doing this part of the examination, but if a child needs a precise and thorough examination, we usually refer the child to an eye expert, an ophthalmologist. Sometimes the ophthalmologist gives the child a sedative medication to ensure the improved view inside the eye that comes from a more relaxed and cooperative child. An ophthalmologist will nearly always use eyedrops to dilate the pupils of the eye, which allows the ophthalmoscope a much better look. We rarely do this for general examinations, however.

EARS, NOSE, AND THROAT

Most parents of small children know that ears are a major concern of pediatricians, primarily because ear infections are so common in early childhood. Since this is such a big part of a child's physical examination, it is worth spending extra time on this aspect so you understand just what doctors are looking for when we shine that light into the ear. It will also help you understand what the doctor is talking about when she tells you what she finds there.

The ear has three components of interest to pediatricians. The *auditory canal* is the tunnel that leads from the outside world back to the eardrum, the *tympanic membrane*. There is a kink in the tunnel, an attribute that protects the ear from damage, so you cannot see the membrane directly. To look at it, the doctor uses an instrument called an *otoscope*. It is a hollow, lighted tube with a magnifying lens. The tapered end of the otoscope straightens out the kink in the auditory canal so the drum is easier to see, although tugging the ear backward a little while inserting the otoscope also helps.

What the doctor usually sees through the otoscope is the translucent eardrum forming a blind alley at the end of the external canal. On the other side of the drum is the middle ear. This tiny cavity contains a chain of minute bones that span the middle ear and transmit sound waves from the vibrating eardrum to the inner ear, where the vibrations are converted to nerve impulses the brain interprets as the sounds we hear. The middle ear has a connecting tube to the back of our throat, the eustachian tube, the job of which is to optimize this process by equalizing the pressure in the middle ear with atmospheric pressure. You can feel this pressure equalize in your own ears when they pop as you go up or down in altitude, such as in an airplane.

Before your doctor inserts the otoscope, however, she will inspect the ear. Severe infection will occasionally make a child's ear stick out at an odd angle. After the doctor has inspected it, she then usually moves the ear, wiggles it a little, because this is an important clue to discovering if there is infection involving the ear canal outside the eardrum. Any discharge or pus in the ear canal—termed *otitis externa*—is evidence of infection there; so-called swimmer's ear is an example of this. Wiggling the ear makes the pain worse for otitis externa but does not affect what is going on behind the eardrum.

The typical toddler ear infection, termed *otitis media*, involves the middle ear, which fills with infected fluid. The pressure from this fluid is responsible for the sometimes intense pain characteristic of otitis media. The infection is caused by bacteria making their way up the eustachian tube from the back of the nose to the middle ear cavity. Sometimes a child has both otitis externa and otitis media if the eardrum has burst from the pressure of the infection in the middle ear and the infected fluid from inside flows out to inflame the ear canal. (Such ruptured eardrums heal without problems.)

As much as anything, skill in examining the middle ear distinguishes the pediatric expert from doctors who have little experience with children. The first evidence of this skill is how the doctor restrains the child for the examination, since virtually no child under three cooperates fully. There are several tricks to doing this well, but all allow the doctor to get a good look at the child's eardrum using the otoscope. A skilled examiner quickly—within seconds—identifies the drum and just as quickly makes a decision about whether it is normal.

For a strong, typically uncooperative toddler, it is usually best to restrain the child on his back on the examination cot, arms above the head. This allows for an effective but quick examination, which is far kinder to the child than allowing him to thrash his head about as he tries to avoid the otoscope. A somewhat more cooperative child can sit on a parent's lap or lean on a shoulder, as the parent holds the child's head still by pressing it against a shoulder. Parents must understand that the otoscopic examination does not hurt your child. It is often better for both the child and the parent if the parent is willing to help hold the child during the ear examination; this reassures both the anxious child and the sometimes equally anxious parent that the procedure really does not hurt.

The eardrum of an infected ear shows distorted landmarks and frequently bulges back at the otoscope light owing to the pressure inside the middle ear. The drum is usually red, but this symptom is not as helpful as is bulging as a sign of infection, because in a crying child, normal drums are often red. Fire engine red drums, however, usually mean infection. Mobility of the eardrum is a key aspect of the examination. If the doctor is unsure about whether there is infection, puffing a little air on the drum through a bulb attached to the side of the otoscope is an excellent way to look for eardrum movement. Infected eardrums do not move normally because of all the fluid behind them.

Children occasionally have fluid behind their eardrums that is not infected, called *serous otitis*. In this situation, the drum is often retracted backward and also does not move normally with an air puff. The drum is not red. Serous otitis is common following an ear infection and often lasts for several weeks or more. It may affect hearing, but usually the child has no ear pain because there is not the intense pressure characteristic of otitis media.

A common problem in examining ears occurs when the ear canals are full of wax, obscuring the eardrum. This wax can be hard to remove, although the experienced ear examiner has several tricks. Wax removal can be frustrating to parents, especially if they have been waiting and waiting to see the doctor, because it can take some time to get the wax out. It is time well spent, though, since a good ear examination is important for most preschool children, especially toddlers.

Examination of a child's nose is uncomplicated. The most common issue is whether there is mucus drainage present and whether this indicates an infection needing antibiotic therapy. Isolated, clear drainage, especially with itchy, watery eyes, can mean an allergy to environmental agents like pollen; the same clear drainage, when accompanied by sore throat, cough, or fever, typically means a viral respiratory infection. We once assumed that cloudy or greenish nose drainage meant there was a sinus infection present needing antibiotics, but recent research has shown this not to be consistently true. Swelling or tenderness next to the nose and under the eyes, however, can mean sinusitis. One other thing the doctor looks for in the nose examination of small babies is flaring outward of the sides of the nose with breathing. Since babies breathe almost exclusively through their noses rather than their mouths, this may be a sign of breathing difficulties.

Every parent knows how important the throat examination is for children. Sticking out the tongue and saying "ahh" is a cliché of medical practice. The reason we ask for that vocalized sound is that it elevates the soft palate—the roof of the throat cavity—out of the way of our line of sight. The wooden stick we use pushes down the tongue, the floor of that cavity. Together these two maneuvers allow us to see what is in the back of the child's throat, particularly the tonsils.

Most parents know from experience that sore throats are an extremely common childhood complaint. Most parents also know that the key distinction to make when evaluating sore throats is whether or not they are "strep" throats, meaning caused by an infection with a bacterium that carries the formal name of *Streptococcus pyogenes*. Strep throats, which need antibiotics, and virally infected throats, which do not, look very similar to the examiner. Both are red, both have enlarged tonsils at the back of the throat, and both can have whitish pus on the tonsils. Research has shown that even experienced examiners cannot tell the two apart. The only way to tell the difference is with a throat culture, a sample taken from a swab rubbed on the back of the throat and sent to the laboratory.

Infants do not get strep throats, but they often get a yeast infection in their mouths called thrush. The infection appears as white patches on the tongue or on the sides of the mouth. At a glance, the patches can just look like milk on the tongue; the key is that they cannot be rubbed off. Thrush can be quite painful to the infant and can interfere with feeding.

NECK

A doctor examining a child's neck is typically looking for swelling, especially in the lymph glands that form two paired chains—one pair running down the front of the neck and one down the back. Swollen or tender lymph glands, especially right under the jaw, are common signs of respiratory infections, both viral ones and those caused by strep. The doctor also assesses how supple the neck is, determining whether the child can flex it forward and nearly touch the chin to the chest. Stiffness of the neck is a key sign of infection around the brain, or *meningitis.*

CHEST AND LUNGS

The chest examination is a particularly important part of a child's physical examination because respiratory ailments are such a common reason for children to see the doctor. As with all the body parts, the chest examination begins with inspection; in this case, the doctor is assessing what we call work of breathing. This is such a key notion in examining children that it is worth pausing to consider it a bit deeper.

The first thing the doctor looks at when assessing work of breathing is how fast the child is breathing—the respiratory rate. This simple observation is very useful in evaluating a child with respiratory complaints because a child with significant lung problems will usually breathe faster than normal. It is so important and so simple to do that your doctor may tell you over the telephone to count the respiratory rate of your own child. Babies in significant distress often breathe at rates of fifty, sixty, or even higher.

The chest cavity containing the lungs is essentially a cage, the bars of which are the ribs. The rigidity of this cage is one of the main things holding a child's lungs open. The cage is covered by several layers of muscles. These layers are arranged in such a way that, when the muscles contract, the volume of the cage increases and the lungs expand. This is *inspiration*, taking in a breath. We get the air out of our lungs, *expiration*, mostly by passive means; the air-expanded chest has enough intrinsic elasticity that when a person stops breathing in, the air leaves on its own, as with a deflating balloon. If a child is using chest muscles to force the air out, that is abnormal; it is a sign of what we call air-trapping in the lungs—the hallmark of asthma.

A child's chest differs from an adult's in an important way. Unlike an adult's, the front part of a child's rib cage is not very rigid because those parts of the ribs are not bone yet—they are still soft cartilage. This has important consequences. If a child's lungs are stiffer than normal, as is common with pneumonia and several other lung conditions, the child often cannot fully expand the lungs. The result is that the chest wall moves the wrong way—inward—when the child takes a breath. Such backward movements of the chest wall are called *retractions*. They are best seen underneath the bottom rib or at the top of the breast bone. Retractions are a sign of increased work of breathing.

After the doctor has inspected your child's chest, the next step is to listen to the breathing with a stethoscope, a tool that has changed little in a century. It is a device that amplifies sounds. Early models were little more than a hollow cylinder the doctor held against the chest, and our current versions are simply updated tubes that do the same thing.

When we use a stethoscope to listen to the lungs, we are checking for several potential abnormalities. Normal breathing consists of an inspiratory phase, breathing in, and an expiratory phase, breathing out. An abnormally prolonged expiratory phase is typical of asthma or other conditions that trap air in the lungs; the child must use chest muscles to squeeze the chest cage and force the air out. The slow-leaving air in this situation often produces a high-pitched musical sound heard through the stethoscope; this is what a doctor calls a *wheeze*.

During the chest examination we also listen for abnormal sounds on inspiration, noises made by air entering the lung. The most important of these is called a *crackle*. Through the stethoscope, crackles sound like someone crinkling up plastic wrap in a ball and then releasing it. Crackles are produced by abnormal fluid in the little air sacs in the lung. In children, they are most characteristic of pneumonia, because lung infection causes fluid to build up in the lung. There are other causes for crackles, but pneumonia is easily the most common in children. If there is a large amount of fluid in the lung or around it, the crackles may be accompanied by diminished breath sounds over the part of the lung with the excess fluid because less air is entering that region.

HEART AND BLOOD VESSELS

The heart is in the middle of the chest, surrounded by the lungs. The key thing to know about how a doctor examines the heart is to realize what the heart is—a pump that moves the blood around our plumbing network of vessels. In fact, the heart is not one pump but two pumps working in series. The right-sided chambers collect oxygen-poor blood from the body and pump it to the lungs to pick up oxygen. The newly oxygenated blood then returns to the left-sided chambers, which pump it out to the rest of the body.

Most parents think of the heart examination as listening to the heart with a stethoscope. Before we do that, however, we can evaluate how well the heart is doing its job both indirectly and directly. The indirect measure of heart function is the degree to which the organs of the body are getting enough oxygen-rich blood to function well. For example, if the kidneys are not getting enough blood flow, the amount of urine a child's body makes in a day will be decreased, something we learn from the child's medical history. Another clue from the history is fatigue. The direct physical examination shows us the effectiveness of the child's circulation; we can feel how strong the pulse is and see how good the circulation is to the skin.

When we listen to a child's heart with a stethoscope, we are listening for several things. What we normally hear are two heart sounds, the "lub" and "dub" of the normal heartbeat. There is usually a longer pause between the "dub" and the "lub" of the next cycle than there is between the two heart sounds, "lub" "dub." Children often have what are called heart *murmurs*. These are the sound of turbulent fluid flowing through the heart. Murmurs are analogous to the sounds you hear in your water pipes as the water flows around kinks in the plumbing system. Since the blood must go through a highly complicated system in the heart, it is not surprising that flow is often turbulent. In addition, a child's chest wall is thin compared to an adult's, making those turbulent regions easy to hear. Most childhood murmurs are normal; we call these innocent murmurs.

Significant murmurs come from some abnormal blood flow pattern in or around the heart, such as an abnormal hole between chambers or a constriction of flow into or out of a chamber. These significant murmurs have a different, usually harsher sound to them, and they are also typically louder than innocent murmurs. Differentiating innocent from significant murmurs is a skill that comes only from extensive experience examining children. If your child's doctor cannot decide if a murmur is significant or not, he will often ask an expert—a cardiologist—to listen to your child's heart. If there is still any question about the murmur, a test called an *echocardiogram* will clarify the issue. You will learn about this test in the next chapter. If your child has a murmur, I encourage you to listen to it with the doctor's help through the stethoscope; it makes it much easier to understand what the doctor is talking about.

ABDOMEN

Abdominal complaints are very common reasons for a child to see the doctor, so the part of the physical examination devoted to the abdominal organs is often a key part of the evaluation. There are many organs in the abdominal cavity, but the most important for our purposes are the liver, the spleen, and the gastrointestinal organs, comprising the stomach and the small and large intestines.

The liver lies in the upper right part of the abdomen. Most of it is tucked up under the rib cage, with less than an inch extending below the last rib, a bit more than an inch in babies. When a person takes a big breath, the diaphragm, which separates the chest cavity from the abdominal cavity, flattens out and pushes the liver down. The examiner uses this fact to feel the lower edge of the liver by asking the patient to take a big breath. The liver edge is not deep within the abdomen—just a half-inch or so beneath the skin—so the examiner feels for it relatively lightly. What the doctor is feeling for is any tenderness or enlargement of the liver. The list of things that can cause these abnormalities in children is a long one, but infection and heart problems are at the top of the list.

The spleen lies on the left side of the abdominal cavity, opposite the liver. Like the liver, it is tucked up under the rib cage. The spleen is normally quite a bit smaller than the liver, however, and usually the examiner cannot feel it at all, even at the end of a deep breath. A doctor's usual assumption is that a child's spleen must be about twice its normal size for it to be felt. An enlarged spleen is most often a sign of infection of some kind. The spleen becomes extremely large and often tender if a child has *infectious mononucleosis* (more commonly called *mono*), a viral infection.

The stomach lies just under the lower end of the breastbone, primarily on the left side of the abdomen and just below the spleen. The small intestine leads out the bottom of the stomach. This long tube, the place where most of our digestion of food happens, is as long as twenty feet in an adult, proportionately less in children. It is coiled in a way that allows it to move around a good deal, something we easily feel happening inside us. The small intestine connects to the large intestine, the colon, in the lower right part of the abdomen. The large intestine is much shorter than the small intestine; it extends across the lower part of the abdomen and then connects to the rectum, and its job is primarily to absorb water.

Hanging off a blind alley of the large intestine, just beyond where the small intestine joins it, is an organ frequently important in pediatric practice—the appendix. The appendix has no function at all, although it may once have been important to humans when our diet was largely plants. Grazing animals, for example, have a huge appendix that is an important part of their digestive system. For humans, the appendix is useless until it causes us trouble, when it becomes worse than useless. Inflammation of the appendix is called *appendicitis*. If an inflamed appendix bursts open into the abdominal cavity, it causes a serious infection called *peritonitis*.

The doctor examines a child's abdomen by touching it, pushing on it, and listening to it with a stethoscope. The best way to do this is to start with light touching and move on to a deeper examination, especially if the child's chief complaint is abdominal pain. One thing the doctor is feeling for is organs—the liver and spleen—and unusual deep swellings, called masses. The doctor also listens to the abdomen to hear the gurgling of the intestines; obstruction of the intestines or inflammation often makes the normal gurgling change in specific ways.

The doctor's abdominal examination of a child with abdominal pain is usually directed, at least initially, to answer one key question: is the pain suspicious for appendicitis or some other condition that would require surgery? The attributes of this kind of pain, not surprisingly termed a surgical abdomen, are that it is localized to one spot and it produces what are called *peritoneal signs*. The *peritoneum* is the lining of the abdominal cavity. An appendix about to burst, or one that already has, inflames the peritoneum, resulting in a specific kind of pain called *rebound tenderness*. This is pain that is worse when the examiner stops pushing and lets the child's abdomen "rebound" back to where it was. Another way to assess rebound is to ask the child to take a few steps or bounce up and down—true rebound tenderness makes a child unwilling or even unable to do this. If the doctor is worried about appendicitis, he will probably order one or more tests (which you will read about in the next chapter) and ask a surgeon to see your child.

By far the most common cause of abdominal pain in children is *gastroenteritis*, the "stomach flu." This is caused by an infection from one of a long list of viruses. Children with this problem often have mildly tender intestines when examined, but unlike appendicitis, the tenderness does not localize to a single spot and there is no rebound tenderness. Children with the flu also usually have vomiting, diarrhea, or both.

A common problem when examining a child's abdomen is that many children are quite ticklish. This can be amusing, but it can also get in the way of doing a good evaluation. There is a standard trick doctors often use to get around this problem. If you have a ticklish child of your own, you can try it out. The examiner usually finds that the ticklishness disappears if he places the child's own hand on the back of his hand, moving when he moves and pushing when he pushes.

GENITALIA

Examination of the genital area is usually not a big part of a child's overall physical examination except for one common condition— diaper rash in infants. Experienced pediatric practitioners have standard ways of deciding if such a rash is caused by simple irritation or infection with either yeast or bacteria. Babies with thrush often also have yeast diaper rash, since both conditions are caused by the same microorganism.

The doctor will also look to see if there are any malformations present. The most common of these is a single testicle in the scrotal sac—an *undescended testicle*. The testicles are formed in the lower abdominal cavity and before birth descend down into the scrotum. Occasionally one of them does not do this normally. If it has not descended by a year or so of age, we use medications or even surgery to correct it. Undescended testicle is usually not a chief complaint because it takes a very astute parent to notice this condition. However, checking for it is a good example of why a complete examination is important; sometimes the doctor finds things important to a child's health that were not anticipated by the history.

EXTREMITIES, JOINTS, AND MUSCULOSKELETAL SYSTEM

These parts of a child's body are among the least mysterious to examine. If there is something wrong with them, the lump, bump, or painful spot is usually readily apparent. The standard things for the doctor to assess are swelling, deformity, tenderness, or limitation of movement. Another important aspect of the examination for any injured arm, leg, hand, or foot is the circulation and sensation below it; swelling and injuries can interfere with the blood vessels and nerves passing through the region to the body parts beyond.

SKIN

Children get a lot of rashes, and evaluation of a rash is a frequent part of a doctor's examination. Diagnosing rashes is one of the arts of medical practice, and a doctor's proficiency at doing that is very much related to experience; identifying rashes is largely a matter of pattern recognition, of seeing something one has seen before. Parents, of course, want the doctor to tell them what their child's rash is from. Pediatricians and family doctors who care for children look at the situation a little differently than parents; we are interested in identifying those rashes that either need treatment or that are signs of serious illness. We know most rashes go away on their own, many of them without our ever knowing their precise cause. Chronic skin problems are cared for by skin experts—dermatologists—and a child with a chronic problem is often best served by a dermatologist.

Skin infections caused by bacterial infections, termed *impetigo*, typically need some form of antibiotic treatment, either an antibiotic cream or an oral medicine. The hallmark of these infections is red inflammation of the underlying skin with some kind of scaling crust on top, which may take the form of blisters filled with white pus. Impetigo commonly occurs on a child's face around the mouth, although any moist area of the skin is prone to it.

Rashes caused by skin inflammation or irritation, *contact dermatitis*, can look similar to impetigo; like impetigo, these types of rashes often have blisters, although usually these blisters are filled with clear fluid rather than cloudy pus. The hallmark of contact dermatitis is itching, often intense itching. The child may scratch the rash so much it becomes infected, turning it into a form of impetigo. Poison ivy or poison oak rash are typical examples of contact dermatitis rashes. The doctor usually treats them with creams, often one containing a corticosteroid medication.

Eczema is a chronic skin problem common in children. It causes a scaling rash most commonly found on the face, the outside of the elbows, or the back of the legs. Eczema often runs in families and is common in children with allergic problems. We have several strategies for treating eczema with anti-inflammatory creams of various kinds, but it usually continues to be a chronic problem throughout childhood.

Many viruses, especially the ones that cause gastroenteritis, come with a rash in addition to other symptoms. These rashes are usually tiny red bumps that do not cause the child any distress. They do not need any special treatment, but their presence is often helpful because it gives us clues about what else is going on.

A final, very common cause of rashes in children is a reaction to medications, particularly antibiotics. These rashes are usually most prominent on the trunk and abdomen. If your child breaks out in a rash several days after starting a medicine, it may be a coincidence, but it also is a good bet that the medicine is causing the rash. If that happens, parents should call their child's doctor.

NERVOUS SYSTEM

The nervous system is usually the last thing the physician examines, however, it is a very important component of the total evaluation. How the doctor examines a child's nervous system is highly dependent upon the age of the child and how cooperative he or she is. The examination is also age-dependent because the doctor looks for different specific things depending upon the age of the child. The evaluation can be fairly cursory, such as for a child in the emergency department with asthma, or it can be extraordinarily detailed, such as for a child who may have suffered a convulsion.

In an infant, the examiner first looks at the state of the child's alertness, the ability to look at and follow a penlight, and general muscle tone. Head circumference relative to the infant's length and weight is important. The doctor will also assess several reflexes babies have but later lose as they grow normally. Older infants and toddlers are assessed on the basis of a series of normal neurological milestones, such as reaching for an object, transferring an object from one hand to another, sitting without support, rolling over, and walking. The doctor will either elicit these actions herself or ask the parent about a child's ability to do them.

The neurological examination of an older child or adolescent proceeds much as it would for an adult. The major components of these exams include level of consciousness and awareness, the sensory nervous system, what the child can feel, and the motor nervous system, an assessment of the major muscle groups in the body. The examination includes testing of a variety of normal reflexes, such as those elicited by tapping tendons with a rubber mallet and observing for muscle twitch. If the doctor has not already done it, a detailed examination of the retina with an ophthalmoscope is an important part of the nervous system evaluation.

Ÿ   Ÿ   Ÿ

As in the previous chapter, I have included here a typical physician recording of a complete physical examination, using as an example the same child with the breathing problems from the last chapter. I have avoided most medical abbreviations, since a typically abbreviation-loaded record can be indecipherable to nonphysicians. Notice that the length of the record is not an accurate measure of how much time the physician spent doing the examination; sometimes the shortest records are the result of a long, meticulous examination.

Vital signs: Temperature 98.8, pulse 88, respiratory rate 40, blood pressure 105/68.

General assessment: Alert-appearing boy in moderate respiratory distress.

Head: Normally formed.

Eyes, ears, nose, throat: No discharge. Visual acuity grossly normal. Pupils equal, round, and normally reactive to light. Ears normal. Throat mildly red, tonsils moderately enlarged without pus.

Neck: Supple with moderately tender and enlarged anterior lymph nodes.

Lungs: Respiratory rate increased at 40. Moderately increased work of breathing with retractions. Auscultation shows prolonged expiratory time with diffuse wheezes throughout both lung fields. Dry cough with deep inspiration.

Heart and blood vessels: Normal sinus rhythm without murmur, pulses normal.

Abdomen: Soft, nontender. No abnormal masses. Liver normal, no spleen felt.

Genitalia: Normal male.

Extremities: Normally formed. No pain or swelling.

Skin: No rash.

Nervous system: Alert and oriented. Motor and sensory normal, reflexes normal.

ꙮ   ꙮ   ꙮ

Most doctors talk to the parent and, if appropriate, to the child during the physical examination. There is a good reason to do this besides just being social; it gives us an opportunity to review salient points of the medical history, even asking the same questions again. Often a parent will think of something of importance the second time a question is asked because our initial conversation gets them mulling things over in their mind. Thus the history can evolve and even change, often in important ways, as a result of communication during the examination process.

I have told you that the secret to an effective physical examination is consistency, doing it the same way every time. Of course, that generalization is not completely true; every doctor modifies the examination as he proceeds, depending on the child's physical findings. For example, if I look in the back of the child's throat and see the huge tonsils characteristic of infection—say, infectious mononucleosis—then I will pay special attention to the abdominal examination when I feel for an enlarged spleen, something also characteristic of that disorder. Or if I find the red eyes and nasal congestion typical for allergies, I will look closely at the child's skin, searching for any signs of eczema. Sometimes I will even go back to the same body part I have already examined for a second look if I encounter something that makes me question my first assessment.

All of us tailor the examination as we go because we are always forming hypotheses about what is wrong with the child and then testing these theories as we proceed. This is only natural. However, it can also be a trap for the physician. It can lead us down preconceived paths. When that happens, we may look only for physical findings that confirm what we expect to find; we can lose our open-minded approach to the physical examination by seeing what we already believe to be the case. A good physician guards against doing that, but it is always a risk. Laboratory tests like blood tests, urine tests, X-rays, and various scans are some of the tools we use to test the hypotheses we are forming about what is wrong with a child. Many diagnoses do not need any kind of testing, but many do. How doctors use the wide variety of tests available to us is the subject of the next chapter.

COMMUNICATION CHECKLIST FOR PARENTS

1. Watch closely while the doctor examines your child.
2. Be ready to help with the examination, especially by reassuring your child.
3. Do not wait to ask about anything the doctor is doing that you do not understand—ask as it is happening.
4. Be ready to elaborate on previous points of your child's history or to answer new questions the doctor might have.
5. If you think of new issues in your child's medical history during the examination that may be important, do not wait—tell the doctor as you think of them.

Chapter 4
SHARP NEEDLES AND COLD X-RAYS
How Doctors Use Common Tests

This chapter concerns the third component of the three-pronged system doctors use to discover how to help your sick or injured child. Once your doctor has completed the history and physical examination, she will consider if there is any need for laboratory testing. This is an enormous topic; doctors have thousands of tests that could typically be used in many situations. In spite of this huge number, however, in most cases we usually rely on a list of tests one could write on less than a single full sheet of paper.

Understanding these common tests and the questions they are designed to help answer is well within the ability of most parents. In the harried and time-pressed setting of many medical encounters, it is a huge advantage to have this sort of understanding. This information will also help make the tests less scary for both parents and children. Of course, we doctors should explain what the tests are for and how they are done, but we do not always do as good a job at this as we should. You will learn about common blood, spinal fluid, urine, and stool tests for children, as well as about X-rays, computed tomographic scans, ultrasound scans, and magnetic resonance imaging scans. Most importantly, you will learn how doctors use these tests to figure out what is wrong with your sick child, and that knowledge will greatly facilitate good communication between you and your child's doctor.

When most people think about how doctors diagnose and treat diseases, they usually think first of the tests, the many sophisticated ways doctors have to look inside the body. More than anything, it is the tests, especially all the scans with their amazing ability to capture images of the inner organs of the body, that define modern medicine. After all, how doctors talk to and examine patients has not changed much in centuries, but the medical tests and equipment we use are evolving constantly into newer and better modalities. Such tests are particularly important when, in spite of a good history and physical examination, a doctor still is not sure what is going on with a child or what to do about it.

Before you read about all these tests, however, you need to understand some important limitations, even dangers, in using them. Surprisingly, the most fundamental danger is not a physical one. Medical tests truly are wonderful tools, but sometimes they *cause* confusion rather than resolve it. I have met many parents who think getting tests of some kind is always part of a thorough examination of their child. Of course, that is not so; the previous two chapters have shown you how, much of the time, a good doctor can figure out what is wrong on the basis of a detailed discussion with you and a careful examination of your child. In fact, it is often the most experienced doctors who order the fewest tests because they have seen so much over the years that their clinical instincts, founded on a decade or two of practice, are all they need most of the time. So if your child's doctor orders a long list of tests, this may not be a good thing. It may mean he has no idea what is going on. If you think this might be the case, ask him; a good doctor will always share what he knows—and what he doesn't know—with you.

There is another key concept you should understand before we get into the details of how specific tests are done and what they mean, and that is the intrinsic error built into the tests themselves. This important principle extends far beyond medicine; it is important to any scientist who measures things, from physicists to oceanographers. Blood test results can serve as a good example to illustrate how the principle applies to medical practice.

When a doctor orders a blood test, for example, a blood count, the blood sample is run through a machine that counts the various kinds of cells and prints out the result. That result will be a number, for example, a cell count of 12,000. (You will read about what that means later in the chapter.) This number, however, is really only an approximate guess of what the child's "true" blood cell count is. It is a close guess, but it is still a guess. In fact, if the doctor drew another blood sample from your child five minutes after the first one and sent it off to the laboratory, the number would not be the same. It would be close, but not the same.

Statisticians deal with this intrinsic error with something they call the *confidence interval*. They define this as the range of values, in our example, from perhaps 11,900 to 12,100, in which they are 95 percent sure the true blood count lies. But we are never totally sure about these things. Although highly unlikely, the true value in our example could be 14,000. All medical tests have similar built-in errors.

Why does this esoteric statistical principle matter to parents sitting with their child in the emergency department? It matters very much, because it means many, even most tests have about a 5 percent chance of being wrong. If the doctor orders lots of tests, say, twenty of them, the chances of one of those results being wrong, or at least being seriously misleading, gets fairly high. And that can be a problem if a wrong test result leads to a wrong conclusion.

What happens more frequently is that a spurious test result leads to more tests, each with built-in error rates of their own, and so on. The medical teaching literature has many examples of what can happen when doctors, in an effort to diagnose a complex case, use a shotgun approach by ordering all manner of tests. The doctor may end up being misled by the results, and sometimes dangerous things can happen to the patient because of it. The best solution to this problem is to make sure that all tests are reasonably connected to the original history and physical examination.

A key point to remember is that it is never a good idea to subject your child to a test just because you or the doctor is curious about the result. All medical tests have risks, even simple blood and urine tests. One of the chief risks is that the test result will not be helpful and, by confusing the doctor, may even be harmful. We doctors often describe this situation as the *risk–benefit ratio*; that is, does the benefit to the child of getting the information from the test far outweigh the risk of doing the test? So it is always a good idea to ask your child's doctor why a particular test is needed and what the doctor will do with the result. With these caveats, we can move on to descriptions of commonly used tests: what they are, how they are done, and what the results usually mean.

BLOOD TESTS

Your two-year-old daughter has had a fever since yesterday, has had progressively less and less to eat or drink, and has been vomiting up the little she did drink. She also seems a little listless to you and less interested in what is going on around her. You call your child's regular doctor, who, after hearing the story, advises you to take your daughter to the emergency room at the hospital. Besides the all-important history and physical examination, the doctor will very likely order some blood tests on your daughter— which ones and why?

A good way to think of all blood tests is that they measure things about one of the two components of the blood: the actual fluid of the blood, termed the *plasma,* or the things floating in the fluid, the blood cells. It is the cells that keep us from seeing through blood; if a glass tube of blood is spun in a centrifuge, sending the cells to the bottom, the fluid above is normally yellowish in color and clear. The child in the example would most likely get both kinds of tests.

The most common test is called the *complete blood count,* or CBC. There are three kinds of cells floating in the blood: *red blood cells, platelets,* and *white blood cells.* The red blood cells are what make blood red, and they are red because they are filled with the pigment hemoglobin. They have one job, which is to carry oxygen and deliver it to the body, and it is the hemoglobin that does the oxygen carrying. A person who does not have enough red blood cells, or whose cells are short on hemoglobin, is called *anemic.* A child with mild anemia will look normal; more severe anemia makes a child look pale. Having too many red blood cells also happens sometimes, but this is uncommon, especially in children.

The platelets are tiny particles, much smaller than red or white cells, that help make the blood clot. Doctors are worried when they see very low platelet counts, especially if a child shows abnormal bleeding. The hallmark of a child who needs a check of platelet count is a peculiar rash of tiny red spots. These show places where there has been bleeding under the skin. High platelet counts happen, too, but that is uncommon.

The blood count parents are most likely to hear about, especially if their child is sick with fever, is the white blood cell count. This is because the main job of white blood cells is to fight infection, so when a child has an infection, the total white count often (but not always) goes up. The white count gets especially high when a child has an infection from bacteria, as compared with infections from viruses. Sometimes, if an infection is particularly severe, the white blood cell count is actually low because all the cells are being used up in the body to fight infection. If the count is too low, this is potentially a serious matter.

White blood cells come in several varieties, and bacterial infection also often causes a shift in the relative proportions of white blood cells circulating in a sick child. The counting of these subtypes of white cells is called the *differential count*, and doctors often use it along with the total white count to decide if a child has a bacterial infection.

The blood cell count is an often-used and important test in situations where a child has a fever mainly because the doctor is trying to decide if the child needs antibiotics. Since antibiotics kill bacteria, the doctor prescribes them if she thinks a child has a bacterial infection. Antibiotics do nothing for a viral infection, so if the total situation suggests that a virus is the culprit, the child usually will not receive them.

What about the noncellular components of the blood? A child like the one in the example has been sick for some time with vomiting, and this can alter the concentrations of some important chemicals and proteins in the blood. The doctor most commonly checks on this possibility with a test called either a *chemistry panel* or an *electrolyte panel*, often abbreviated as BMP (for basic metabolic profile) or lyte panel. The components of the usual blood chemistry panel are these: glucose (blood sugar), sodium, potassium, chloride, bicarbonate ion, creatinine, and urea nitrogen. Sometimes the doctor will add the measurement of several proteins made by the liver to the chemistry profile if she is concerned if the child's liver is working normally. These are called *liver function tests* (abbreviated LFTs) or sometimes a liver panel. Their values go up if the liver is inflamed in some way.

What a parent should know about the chemistry panel is that the doctor most commonly uses it to tell if a child is dehydrated and if the kidneys are working well. An abnormal chemistry panel often shows that a child needs intravenous fluid therapy or even needs to be admitted to the hospital. Together the CBC and chemistry panel are by far the most common blood tests doctors use for children. This is particularly so in the setting of a walk-in acute-care clinic or emergency department.

If your child were the one in the example, how would these tests be done and how much blood would have to be taken? No one enjoys being stuck with a sharp needle, but this is a particularly important question for parents of uncomprehending children. In general, doctors can get a blood sample in one of three ways: from a vein, from an artery (rarely done), or from the tissue itself—called a *capillary* sample. Most times we use a vein, usually the one in the crease of the elbow.

A technician from the laboratory usually does the actual blood drawing. This is not easy when dealing with a small, struggling child, and doing it well takes considerable practice and experience. It is always appropriate for a parent to ask the technician how experienced she is in drawing blood from children; if you are concerned, ask for the most experienced person available.

Good blood-drawing skills are particularly important when a technician is taking a sample for a CBC. This is because the blood to be tested goes in a special tube containing a chemical that keeps the blood from clotting. Since the blood cells are what the test measures, any small clots in the tube trap the cells in them and confuse the machinery doing the test. The practical effect of this is that the blood needs to flow quickly and easily from the child's vein, out through the needle, and into the collecting syringe; if the technician needs to poke and prod too much, the blood will clot. Small clots are hard to see in the sample, so often we do not know this has happened until the laboratory calls back and tells us the sample is no good. This is always bad news, since it means the child needs to have a fresh needle stick. If this happens to your child, understand that it is an unfortunate complication of children having little veins that are hard to find.

It is also appropriate for a parent to ask if anything can be done to reduce the pain from the needle stick. We now have several creams available that numb the skin and reduce the pain from the needle, the most common of which is called *EMLA*. However, these creams do take time to work, typically about an hour, so their benefits must be weighed against the need to delay the test until the child is comfortable. Properly used, these creams do reduce the pain. Keep in mind, though, that a good portion of a toddler's discomfort in getting a blood test is from a strange person leaning over them and holding their arm tightly. The application of EMLA will not help that; only a reassuring parent and a skilled technician can.

How much blood is needed for cell counts and chemistries? Until recently, children were at a disadvantage because the makers of laboratory machinery did not take children's needs into account. This has changed dramatically in the past decade, and now most of the common blood tests can be done using small amounts of blood. These days, a complete blood count, differential count, and serum chemistry panel can all be done on about a half teaspoon of blood (two to three milliliters).

Another blood test doctors often perform on children sick with fever is a *blood culture*. Doctors do this test when they are worried a child might have bacteria present in the bloodstream. This represents a serious infection by itself, but it also can lead to worse problems if not diagnosed and treated. The child in the example—the two-year-old with the fever and lethargy—would most likely need a blood culture. If a doctor is concerned enough about a possible infection, called *sepsis* or *bacteremia*, she will usually give a child antibiotics to treat it while waiting for the result of the blood culture, which takes several days to complete. Parents may wonder why the test takes several days. A laboratory technician puts a small blood sample (usually another half a teaspoon or so) into a special culture bottle containing food for the bacteria; if bacteria are in the sample, they will multiply and become obvious, a process which takes time.

Of course, there are many, many blood tests besides these that doctors order for children. Most of the time, however, any additional tests do not replace the basic ones but are added to them because the CBC and blood chemistries are excellent screening tests for serious illness. It is always appropriate, and also just good practice, for parents to ask the doctor specifically what blood tests are being done and the rationale for them.

SPINAL FLUID TESTS

Your five-week-old baby has been fussy for a day and is nursing less and less well. Today she seems listless, and you have had to wake her up for her last two feedings. When you do so again, she feels warm and you take her temperature—it is 102 degrees. You call your pediatrician's office, and his nurse tells you to take your baby to the hospital emergency department as soon as possible. Worriedly, you do so. Why was your pediatrician so concerned? What tests will the doctor do?

An infant with a fever is a common problem in pediatrics and there is an accepted, standard way to evaluate and treat such a problem. The main concern is for bacterial infection, which can rapidly become overwhelming in infants because their infection-fighting immune system has not yet matured. If the doctor waits to do anything until the signs of potential infection besides fever are obvious, things like shock and decreased breathing, it may be too late for the baby. Even though the risk of that happening is low, it is still too high to be ignored, so doctors are aggressive in their testing in this situation.

Virtually all infants with significant fever need a series of tests for bacterial infection. Bacteria circulating in an infant's bloodstream can be spread to other places in the body; a common place is the *meninges*, the membrane that covers the surface of the brain. Infection of the meninges is called *meningitis*. So, an infant who might have this needs not only blood and urine tests but also a procedure known as a *lumbar puncture*—a spinal tap.

Older children sometimes need spinal taps, too, usually because the doctor is concerned about the possibility of meningitis. The listless toddler with fever in the first case, for example, could well need this test. There are other reasons for doing the tap, but by far the most common reason is to look for meningitis. Since children account for the majority of all cases of meningitis, doing a spinal tap is a common pediatric procedure. In fact, a typical pediatric emergency department will do at least several of these each day.

How will a spinal tap tell the doctor if a child has meningitis? The brain floats inside the skull, bathed in and surrounded by *cerebrospinal fluid*, or CSF. This same fluid flows down around the spinal cord, which is contained in a fibrous sac. The sac extends inside the backbone all the way down to the pelvic bone, well below the point where the spinal cord itself ends. This fortunate circumstance allows us to sample easily and safely the same fluid that is flowing over the brain and the meninges. If there is infection in the brain, signs of it will show in the fluid the doctor takes from the lower reaches of the sac.

Spinal taps are not done by technicians; they are done by physicians or rarely by specially trained physician assistants or nurses. The key to success in obtaining CSF is proper positioning of the child. If your child needs a tap, the doctor will lay your child on her right or left side, depending upon preference, and have an assistant curl her up in a ball with chin down and knees up (sometimes infants are supported leaning forward in a sitting position). This opens up a path between the *vertebrae*, the bones in the spinal column, and the fluid-filled sac. The doctor pushes a needle through the skin and along that path into the sac, well below the place were

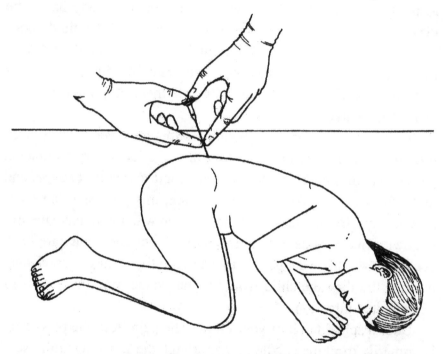

This figure shows how a spinal tap is done. After numbing the child's skin, the doctor inserts the needle in the middle of the back just above the tailbone and slowly advances it at an angle aiming at the child's belly button until it reaches the space containing the spinal fluid. The doctor then collects the fluid into a tube as it drips out. (from Ronald A. Dieckmann, Debra H. Fiser, and Steven M. Selbst, eds., *Pediatric Emergency and Critical Care Procedures* [St. Louis, MO: Mosby-Yearbook, 1997], p. 534, used by permission of Elsevier Health.)

the spinal cord itself has stopped. The CSF then drips out on its own, and the doctor collects it in a tube. The entire procedure usually takes about fifteen minutes, sometimes a little longer. Figure 1 illustrates how it is done on an older child.

What does the doctor do with the CSF, and how long must parents wait for the results? The possibility of meningitis is a serious one, so a technician in the laboratory analyzes the CSF as quickly as possible. Normal CSF is clear, so the doctor already has some idea that there might be an infection present if the fluid looks cloudy when it comes out. Within an hour, the doctor should have the preliminary results, the most important of which is whether there are abnormal cells in the fluid. If there are, some form of meningitis is likely.

The only way to be sure about infection, however, is a CSF *culture*. It resembles the blood culture in that a laboratory technician places a small sample of CSF on a rich food source for bacteria and looks for growth. Like the blood culture, this process often takes several days. Doctors usually treat children who might have meningitis with intravenous antibiotics until the culture results are back because it would be dangerous to wait until the culture is confirmed positive; by then the child would be far worse from the effects of an untreated infection.

Does a spinal tap hurt your child? The pain from the procedure is primarily from the needle going through the skin—a similar sensation to having blood drawn—and like a blood draw, the pain can be helped by using the same EMLA cream to numb the skin as for blood tests. The doctor can also inject into the area a little numbing medication of the sort dentists use. The actual needle used to do the spinal tap is about the same size as the needle used to draw blood. The most upsetting thing about a spinal tap for many children, especially toddlers, is being rolled into a ball to have it done. Parents can help by comforting and reassuring their child. Because the child is lying on his side, facing away from the person doing the tap, a parent can sit closely with the child, looking into his face.

Is the procedure safe? The notion of a spinal tap is frightening to many parents. After all, the whole idea sounds dangerous. There are a good number of urban legends circulating about people injured by a spinal tap; I have heard some of these over my thirty years of pediatric practice. I have never encountered such a situation, however, and the medical literature shows that lumbar punctures done in the setting of this example case are extremely safe. The main problems are some oozing of blood from the needle puncture, which is easy to stop, and sometimes among older children a headache, although this is more common in adults after a spinal tap.

Because a spinal tap is a medical procedure, parents are usually asked to sign a standard consent form. These forms can be frightening to read because they are used to consent to everything from a spinal tap to a heart transplant; the doctor typically fills in the blank at the top of the form listing the particular procedure. Parents should take this opportunity to ask who will be doing the tap and how experienced that person is with children, because experience is crucial for doing it smoothly, and whether they can watch the procedure if they desire, and when they can expect to learn the results of the initial CSF tests.

URINE TESTS

Your five-year-old daughter has been complaining that it hurts to urinate. She has not had any fever, but she complains of vague abdominal pain, her appetite is down, and she has vomited once or twice. Meanwhile, your fourteen-year-old son, a daredevil on his bicycle, tells you his urine has been pinkish in color since he hit a curb and went over his handlebars yesterday and landed on the pavement. You bring both of them to the hospital emergency department. What tests will the doctor there do to evaluate these two problems?

As is the case with blood tests, there are many ways doctors can test urine, but two kinds of urine studies account for the large majority of situations. The most common of these is aptly named the *urinalysis*, abbreviated as UA. Also like blood tests, the urinalysis examines both microscopic particles suspended in the urine, such as cells or bacteria, and the substances in the fluid component of the urine, such as glucose and protein.

The urinalysis is an easily obtained and useful test for the doctor to see if there is anything wrong with a child's urinary tract. Normal urine has virtually no cells in it. If the kidneys or bladder are inflamed for some reason, the urine usually contains white blood cells, red blood cells, or both. If those cells are there, though, the doctor often needs to move on to other, more specific tests of both urine and blood to figure out why.

Other components of the urinalysis include checking for the presence of glucose or protein in the urine (neither should be there) and measuring how concentrated the urine is. The last, coupled with the blood electrolyte panel, is a good way to determine dehydration in a child.

Unlike blood tests, urinalysis is a very easy test to do because all that is needed is for a toilet-trained child to urinate into a container. For children still in diapers, the urine can be collected simply by sticking a small plastic bag around the child's urinary opening (it works for both boys and girls), closing the diaper back up, and waiting. The laboratory only needs a tablespoon of urine to do the test.

The fourteen-year-old boy in the example above who fell off his bike would first get a urinalysis, although since he complained of discolored urine, the doctor would also probably do the simple, age-old test of just holding the urine up to the light and looking at it. If there was visible blood in the boy's urine, however, the urinalysis would still be helpful because it would determine how much blood was there and if anything else was wrong. Afterward the doctor would move on to one of several tests that image or scan the kidneys to see if the boy bruised them. You will read about these tests later in the chapter.

The five-year-old girl in the example most likely has an infection of her urinary tract. The best test for this, for finding bacteria in the urine, is placing the urine in a laboratory incubator. As with the blood and CSF cultures, for a *urine culture*, a technician puts a small urine sample on a rich food source for bacteria and then checks the next day to see if any bacteria are growing. If bacteria are there, the laboratory does some additional tests to identify what kind they are and which antibiotic is best suited to kill them. This is called a *sensitivity test* because it tests to which antibiotics the bacteria are sensitive.

Unfortunately, getting urine for a culture is much more involved and more potentially uncomfortable for the child than getting urine for urinalysis. There are some tests in the urinalysis that can suggest whether the child has an infection, and doctors are sometimes tempted to use these to make the decision, but such tests are unreliable. The gold standard is a urine culture.

The problematic issue is that urine for culture must be sterile, and the skin where the urine comes out, the *urethral meatus*, is loaded with bacteria. So just urinating in a cup or collecting urine in a bag will always yield a sample contaminated with skin bacteria, and the doctor will therefore not know if there really is an infection present. Doctors solve this problem in one of two ways. The first is to collect what is called a *midstream* or *clean catch* sample. To get this test, the area around the meatus is cleaned with antiseptic soap. The child is then asked to start to urinate, and a sample is obtained after the urinary stream has started. The idea is that the contaminating bacteria get washed away and the urine collected in "midstream" will more accurately reflect what is going on inside the child's urinary tract. Doing this, of course, requires a cooperative child who is toilet-trained.

The only way to get uncontaminated urine from a younger child is to place a tiny sterile tube up through the child's urethral meatus and on into the bladder. Called a *urinary catheterization*, it is uncomfortable, even painful for the child. Because of this, it is a test a doctor should not order lightly. However, urinary tract infections, although not as common among children as they are among adults, carry significant implications. Therefore, a child who contracts one, particularly a boy, needs further tests to make sure the kidneys and bladder are normal. So, in spite of the discomfort catheterization may cause a small child, this procedure provides key information for the doctor if the history suggests infected urine.

STOOL TESTS

Your six-month-old child has had ten stools each day over the last two days. He has not had any fever and he seems to feel well, but you are concerned that he might need treatment for the diarrhea. You also worry he is getting dehydrated, so you take him to a walk-in clinic near your home. What tests, if any, will the doctor order for your child?

Most parents of small children have experience with diarrhea—it is a common ailment, particularly among infants and toddlers. Most times it represents a self-limited viral infection or perhaps feeding intolerance, but there are some kinds of diarrhea that are more serious, and we have tests to check for those.

One potential cause is *rotavirus*. There is no specific treatment for this infection, although there is a new vaccine to prevent it.

Rotavirus is highly infectious for other children, and the diarrhea it causes is often quite severe, so it is important to know if it is present. Bacterial intestinal infections, or *dysentery*, were once quite common in America and continue to be common in the third world. Such infections do still occur in this country occasionally. If your child has diarrhea with high fever, bloody stools, and severe pain, the doctor may suspect one of these more severe causes of diarrhea.

Doctors use tests on the child's stool to look for these intestinal infections. Stool tests are the easiest of all tests because the doctor needs only a stool sample in a diaper or container, and children with diarrhea readily provide this. The laboratory then analyzes the stool to look for blood cells, rotavirus, specific disease-causing bacteria, or even intestinal parasites like worms. Children with severe diarrhea can get dehydrated from fluid lost in their stools, so doctors often need to do blood chemistry tests as well to check for that possibility.

X-RAY TESTS

Your ten-year-old child has been sick for three days with a cough. At first the cough was dry, but over the last twelve hours he has started to cough up quite a bit of phlegm. He also has a fever and seems to be breathing faster than normal. He complains of sharp pains in his chest when he takes a deep breath or when he coughs. You are worried he has pneumonia, so you take him to the hospital emergency department.

Meanwhile, and most unluckily for you, your eight-month-old son has been vomiting for almost a day. When you change his diaper, his abdomen looks swollen and you find some bloody mucus in his diaper. You are concerned that something is very wrong in his intestines, perhaps a blockage of some kind, so you take him along with his brother to the emergency department. How will the doctor evaluate your children's problems?

The doctor should, of course, take a careful history from you about what has been happening with your children and do a thorough physical examination, but in both these cases she will likely need more information in the form of X-rays. These are very common tests, so it is a good idea for parents to understand both how X-rays work and how a doctor interprets them. Many parents also have questions about the long-term safety of X-rays: are X-rays harmless, or can they pose a risk to your child?

X-rays, discovered just over a century ago, are electromagnetic energy waves that can pass through many common objects, including our bodies. The different tissues in the body absorb the rays to varying degrees; bone absorbs most of them, air hardly at all, and soft tissues somewhere in between. A photographic film on one side of the child records which rays pass through from the machine on the other side of the child. As a result, bone appears on the film as nearly white because little radiation passes through it, and normal lungs appear nearly black because they are mostly filled with air and thus allow most of the rays through. The actual X-ray image was for many years recorded on a large piece of film that the doctor held up to a light box to read; now virtually all X-rays are recorded by a computer and the images are displayed on a computer screen. Soon after X-rays were discovered, doctors devised ways to increase the number of things they could look at with their new tool, chiefly by using what is called *contrast*—substances that absorb the rays and can be placed in various body structures to highlight them.

One of the most common X-ray tests done on children is the chest X-ray, typically used to see if the child has pneumonia. An experienced doctor can often diagnose pneumonia by listening to a child's chest with a stethoscope, especially if that all-important his-

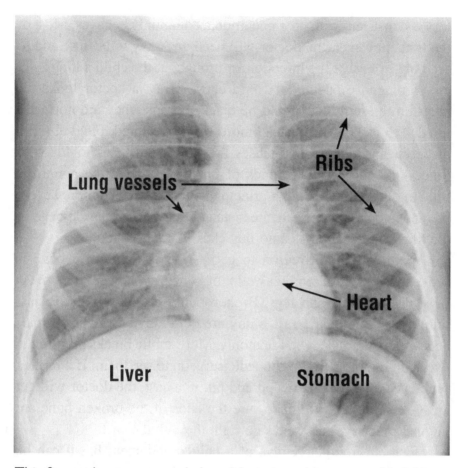

This figure shows a normal chest X-ray in a three-year-old child. To get a good view of the lungs, the child's arms are raised above his head; a parent is frequently asked by the technician to help by doing this while the picture is taken. The lung fields, normally dark because they are mostly air, have several white areas superimposed on them. These include the heart, normal blood vessels inside the lungs, and the ribs. Below the lungs are the liver and the stomach; the former is white because it is solid, the latter is dark because it is full of air. (© CentraCare, used by permission)

tory is consistent with how pneumonia commonly behaves. Most of the time, however, the doctor will need an X-ray to be sure and to see how extensive the infection is throughout the child's lungs.

To diagnose pneumonia on a chest X-ray, a doctor looks for areas on the film that should be black (because they are normally filled with air) but are instead more whitish-colored. Fluid absorbs the rays, and pneumonia causes the lung's airspaces to fill with fluid. Although different kinds of pneumonia have the abnormal fluid in different places, the principle is the same. The more severe the pneumonia, the more white instead of black the lungs appear on the film. Figure 2 shows a normal chest X-ray in a toddler.

Another common reason to get X-rays is to see if a bone is broken. Active children break a lot of bones, so they get a lot of X-rays of their arms and legs. Broken bones are among the easiest things to spot on an X-ray. Many are quite obvious, even for parents with no knowledge of anatomy. More subtle breaks require the eyes of a radiologist or orthopedic surgeon to see them. If a broken limb needs to be straightened and put in a cast, the doctor will get an X-ray afterward to make sure the ends of the broken bone are aligned properly; the X-rays go right through the cast.

Doctors often get X-rays of a child's abdomen, but it can be hard to tell very much about the abdominal organs because they are mostly soft tissue. But if we put a liquid contrast material that absorbs all X-rays inside the intestines, then the areas with the contrast will appear totally white on the film and will show both the boundaries of the intestinal wall and if there is something inside the intestinal cavity that should not be there. This contrast material can be swallowed, after which it reveals the stomach and upper small intestine, or inserted into the large intestine through the rectum. The former test is called a *barium swallow*, the latter is called a *barium enema*. The child with the vomiting and bloody stools would most likely first get a plain abdominal X-ray, followed by barium studies, because his history suggests he may have a blockage in his intestines.

Doctors do a lot of X-rays on children. Is there a risk to a child's health, or are X-rays completely safe? The answer, for chest and abdominal X-rays, is that they are very, very, very safe, but not totally risk-free. All of us are constantly exposed to radiation similar to X-rays. It comes primarily from naturally occurring radioactive matter around us, such as radon gas seeping up through the ground, or from space in the form of cosmic rays. People living at higher altitudes receive higher doses of such background radiation, amounting to about half again as much for someone living on the Colorado plateau compared with someone at sea level. To put things in perspective, the radiation dose in a single chest X-ray, on average, is similar to the background radiation most of us receive during a ten-day time span living our normal lives.

There are several important things to remember about radiation risks. High radiation doses definitely cause death and disease (primarily cancer); the atomic bomb and the disaster at Chernobyl clearly showed this. A second key point is that radiation risk is cumulative over a lifetime. This is an important consideration in caring for children, since they have most of their life ahead of them. Children are also more sensitive to the effects of X-rays than are adults. Still, it is logical to think of routine chest and abdomen X-rays as being virtually without risk unless the child has already received a large radiation dose in the past. If an adolescent girl of childbearing age needs an abdominal X-ray, it is important to make sure she is not in the early stages of pregnancy, since X-rays can harm an embryo. If your teenaged daughter needs an abdominal X-ray, be prepared for that question from the radiology technician.

The actual machine that takes an X-ray is much like a camera with an average shutter speed. Anyone who photographs children knows it is often hard to get them to sit still for a picture. The same is true for X-rays; if the child is moving when the technician trips the switch, the image will be blurred, just as a photograph would be. This is a common problem with chest X-rays in small children. It is relatively easy to hold an arm or a leg still, but a good chest X-ray requires that the film be snapped when the child has taken a deep breath to inflate the lungs fully. X-ray technicians are experienced in doing this, but it can be a challenge to catch a child at the instant of full inspiration. If your toddler needs a chest X-ray, the technician will likely check the quality of the image before you leave the radiology department. Do not be surprised if a second try is needed.

If your small child needs an X-ray, it often helps if you are in the X-ray room, holding the child, talking to him, or both. If you do this with your child, the technician should give you a protective apron to block any wayward X-rays from hitting you. If you are a woman, the technician will probably ask you if you could be pregnant. If you could be, it is especially important for you to wear the apron or even step out of the room when the technician takes the picture.

Sometimes the doctor will order a portable X-ray. These are done with a rolling machine that has an extendable arm holding the X-ray source. Portable X-rays are often not as high-quality as the films taken in the radiology department, but sometimes a child cannot travel to the department for one reason or another. If you stay beside your child when the portable shot is taken—and that is usually a good thing unless you could be pregnant—the technician should give you and anyone else in the room a protective apron to wear.

COMPUTED TOMOGRAPHIC (CT) SCANS

Your son is climbing the tree in your backyard one Saturday afternoon. You see him fall out and whack his head hard on the ground. You run out to him and find him to be a little groggy but conver-

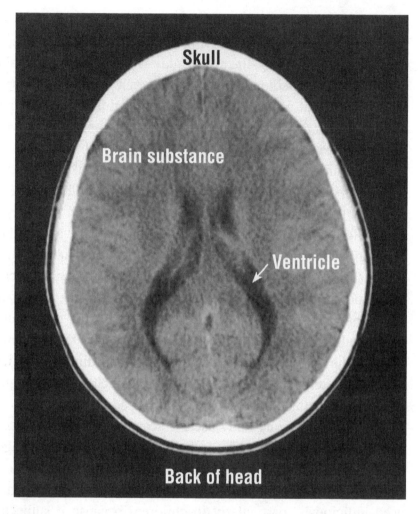

This figure shows one view, or slice, from a CT scan of a normal sixteen-year-old boy's head. The level of this slice is just above the ears and it runs parallel to the ground. The front of the child's head is at the top of the image. The skull bone is white and completely surrounds the brain. The brain itself is hollow, with fluid-filled ventricles inside. You can see that the brain is composed of both *white matter* and *gray matter*, indicated by the different shades of material within the brain substance. (© CentraCare, used by permission)

sant. You scold him for climbing so high in the tree; he responds that he cannot remember climbing the tree at all. Meanwhile, your other son has been sick since yesterday with vague abdominal pain and decreased appetite. Today he has a fever, the pain is worse, and he refuses to eat or drink anything. You load both boys in the car and take them to the hospital emergency department. How will the doctor evaluate them?

Following the usual careful history and physical examination, it is likely that the doctor will order CT scans for both of your sons. A computed topographic scan is a specialized form of X-ray test. The child lies on a platform that is incrementally advanced into the circular scanner. As the child passes through the machine, thin X-ray beams pass from one side of the scanner through the child's body and are detected on the other side of the scanner. By rotating the scanner and detector in a circle, and then using a computer to analyze all the information about how much of the X-ray beams got through the various regions of the body, a two-dimensional image of each incremental body "slice" can be constructed. Figure 3 shows such a single slice from a child's head CT scan.

Doctors most commonly use CT scans to look at the head, the chest, and the abdomen. The technology produces good images of the organs inside those body regions, and the machine has revolutionized how medicine and surgery are practiced. But CT must be used judiciously, particularly in children, because it subjects the child to much more radiation than does a simple chest or abdomen X-ray—two hundred to six hundred times more, depending upon the particular technique used. So if a chest X-ray is the equivalent of ten days of background radiation exposure, a child getting a CT scan receives the same radiation dose as anywhere from fifteen to thirty years of normal living.

The future cancer risk to a child from a single CT scan is still small, and the benefits of getting the information the CT provides nearly always outweigh this tiny risk. However, this may not be the case for children who get many CT scans or who have been exposed to other radiation in the past. Fortunately, this is a relatively small number of children.

The first child in the example, the one who fell out of the tree, probably has a concussion like Sean, our patient in chapter 1. It is common for a child with a concussion to forget what happened during the accident and also during the few minutes before it. The doctor in the emergency department will likely be concerned that, in addition, the boy may have suffered a bruise on the surface of his brain or have other bleeding inside his skull. The quick way to allay those concerns is with a CT scan of the head. Head CT is highly accurate at diagnosing brain injury or skull fractures. It is the most common type of CT scan doctors use, and a typical busy emergency department will account for many of these each day.

The second child in the example, the one with the abdominal pain, would very likely need an abdominal CT scan. The key question the test will answer is whether the child's problem will require operation, such as appendicitis requiring an appendectomy. Abdominal CT scans are often done with two kinds of contrast: oral contrast the child swallows, and intravenous contrast the radiologist injects into the child's bloodstream. Unlike ordinary abdominal X-rays, contrasted abdominal CT scans give an excellent picture of what is going on inside the abdomen. Since the doctor's question is frequently whether the child needs an operation, the tiny radiation risk of the CT far outweighs the value of finding out the correct answer to that question.

CT scanners have gotten much faster over the years, but it still takes several minutes at least to complete a scan, during which time the child must lie still enough to obtain clear pictures. This is frequently a problem with small children, especially toddlers. The scan does not hurt in any way, but the child must lie still. For this reason, young children are often given some sort of sedative medication to make them sufficiently drowsy to cooperate. The risks of doing this are minimal, but they are not zero.

The main risk is that the drugs will sedate the child so much that breathing may slow down to dangerous levels. Doctors have standard ways to watch for this and deal with it if it happens. At a minimum, the child should wear a lighted probe on the finger or toe to measure blood oxygen level, and the child may need to breathe some extra oxygen until the effects of the drugs wear off. The child typically needs an intravenous line, too, both for the contrast injection and sometimes for sedative drugs.

ULTRASOUND SCANS

Your nine-year-old daughter has had pain in her right flank for a day and has not felt like eating anything. She had a urinary tract infection the previous year, and you are worried she might have another one, so you take her to the emergency department. What tests will the doctor order?

The first thing the doctor will do is probably a urinalysis and urine culture test as you read about earlier in this chapter, but it is also quite likely your daughter will receive a *kidney ultrasound test*. Doctors frequently use ultrasound technology on children. These scans do not provide the fine detail of CT scans, but unlike CT they are completely risk-free, except for the general cautions at the beginning of this chapter about using and interpreting information from any medical test. Ultrasound tests do not hurt. Unlike the situation for CT scans, the child can be moving around some during the test, so there is rarely any need for sedative drugs.

Ultrasound works using the same principles as sonar in a submarine and the way whales and dolphins navigate. First, the technician puts a spot of jelly on the skin so there is good contact with the ultrasound probe and then she touches the probe to the child's skin, often aiming it in different directions. The probe itself emits high-frequency sound waves, inaudible to us, that travel through the tissue. When these waves strike a boundary, as between two organs, some of the waves are reflected back to the probe while others keep going. These strike other boundaries, reflect back a portion of the waves, and so on until the strength of the waves dies out. The result is a two-dimensional image on a screen in real time; that is, the operator can get key information and make measurements, such as how big a child's kidney is, as the scan is being done.

Ultrasound works best for structures that have various kinds of liquids in them, such as tissues, blood vessels, and organs like the liver and the kidney. Obstetricians have long used ultrasound to see how a baby is growing inside the mother's uterus. Heart doctors, especially pediatric ones, are also frequent ultrasound users, in which case the test is called an *echocardiogram*. It is an excellent tool for studying the heart, especially because the cardiologist can make a video of it beating in real time. Another common use is with premature babies. These infants have very thin skull bones and large soft spots, so ultrasound gives a very good image of their brains.

If your child needs an ultrasound, it is usually because the doctor wants to check the kidneys, liver, or other organs in the abdomen. It also is a good test for checking blood flow into and out of those organs. There really is no downside to using ultrasound to image a child's abdomen, and doctors frequently do this test before any others to see if they can get enough useful information from it to avoid the need for the more complicated CT scan.

MAGNETIC RESONANCE IMAGING (MRI) SCANS

Your energetic son, the one who previously flipped his bicycle and bruised his kidney, is also an avid snowboarder. He turns the wrong way going through the half-pipe and twists his knee. He keeps going the rest of the afternoon, but the next day his knee is swollen and he cannot bear much weight on it. You call your child's doctor, who refers you to an orthopedic surgeon. How will the surgeon evaluate your son's knee?

The orthopedist will first examine the knee, of course, although sometimes the swelling makes it difficult for the surgeon to be sure of the exact nature of the injury. In that case, your son may just wear a knee brace for a few days until the swelling goes down, but it is becoming more and more common for injuries like this to be evaluated with an MRI scan, a test that gives exquisite, finely detailed pictures of many parts of the body, including the knee.

How ultrasound and CT work is complicated; how MRI works is *very* complicated. For our purposes, it is enough to understand that MRI uses a giant magnet surrounding a long tube, into which the child slides on a special table. The magnet, in effect, makes the hydrogen atoms in the body line up in accordance with the magnetic field. The machine then delivers pulses of radio waves that change this atomic orientation, making them spin in different ways, and measures what happens when the pulses are turned on and off. A sophisticated computer system then converts this information into an image, using the fact that different tissues respond to the pulses in different ways. The great advantages of MRI are that the images show whatever is scanned in astonishing detail, and unlike X-rays, no radiation is involved. The images are displayed as slices through the body, as with the CT scan. Figure 4 shows one such MRI slice of a child's head.

MRI does have problems, especially when used with children.

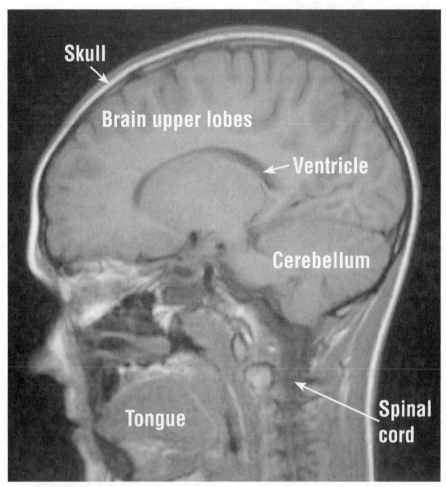

This figure shows a single slice from a normal child's MRI scan. Its orientation is perpendicular to the CT scan image in figure 3. The extraordinary detail of MRI technology clearly shows the child's mouth, lips, and nose. You can see the white and gray matter in the upper lobes of the brain, as well as the *cerebellum*, the portion of the brain that controls balance, a side view of a ventricle, and what is called the mid-brain. You can also see much besides the brain, including the tongue and the spinal cord, which emerges from the bottom of the brain. (© CentraCare, used by permission)

One problem is that, although CT requires the child to lie still for a time, MRI requires the child to lie very still for a very much longer time, often an hour or more. For this reason, children are often deeply sedated for MRI scanning. Such deep sedation carries risks, particularly that of decreased breathing. Sometimes the sedation needs to be so deep that the services of an anesthesiologist are needed because the child is essentially anesthetized as for a surgical operation.

If a child is old enough to cooperate with the MRI, as was the snowboarder in our example, having an MRI is still not a pleasant experience. Many people become claustrophobic when they are inside the long tunnel of the magnet, although the newest generation of scanners is more open. The MRI machine also is loud, so loud that ear plugs or totally muffling headphones are needed both for the patient and anyone else in the room. Finally, nothing metal can be near the magnet.

In spite of these issues, MRI is fast becoming the definitive way to look inside the human body, particularly the brain. If your child's doctor really needs to know what is in there, MRI is the test to do. In fact, MRI provides so much anatomical detail that medical educators are concerned that today's medical students are not learning to polish their physical examination skills. If you or your child ever has an MRI, ask to see the images—they are spectacular.

ELECTROCARDIOGRAM (ECG) TESTS

The electrocardiogram is an extremely common test doctors perform on adults, particularly those with heart problems; it is the cornerstone of diagnosing heart attacks. The ECG is much less commonly done on children, but now and then a child needs one.

As you have read, the heart is a pump, its chambers filled with blood. The walls of the chambers are solid muscle; when the heart muscle contracts, blood is pumped around the body. Like all muscles, the signal for the heart muscle to contract is an electrical one. It comes down from the heart's pacemaker and courses down a series of conducting fibers that are much like wires. The ECG measures how the electrical signal to the heart muscle is moving down the fibers and spreading out through all the muscle fibers.

An ECG does not hurt a child, and it is relatively fast and easy to do. The technician attaches some small electrodes to the child's wrists, ankles, and in a line across the child's chest. Once the electrodes are in place, the machine only takes a minute or so to record the tracings on a large piece of graph paper.

The experts at reading ECGs are cardiologists, although any doctor who cares for children can look at the paper tracing and glean important information. These days there are computer programs built into the machine that do an excellent job at scanning and reading the ECG results immediately. So, most times, the doctor finds out the answer on the spot.

ELECTROENCEPHALOGRAM (EEG) TESTS

Sometimes called a brain wave test, the EEG measures the electrical activity on the surface of the brain, the *cortex*. Like our hearts, our brains use electricity. In fact, the brain actually runs on electricity, on current produced by the chemical reactions within the brain cells as they communicate with one another. Doctors use the EEG to decide if a child has a seizure problem, because seizures consist of disorganized electrical discharges in the cortex. A child with an ongoing seizure has a wildly abnormal EEG, but often a child with a seizure tendency will have an identifiable abnormal spot, a *seizure focus*, that we can see on the EEG even in the absence of an active seizure.

Seizures, or convulsions, are not uncommon in children. Most times we can tell if an older child or adult is having a seizure just by looking at them; usually they will have involuntary twitching movements of the eyes, arms, or legs. Often the person becomes unresponsive or unconscious as well. Small children, particularly infants, are different; it can be very difficult to tell if they are having a seizure. All manner of odd-looking spells, such as staring vacantly into space, arching or twisting the body, or sudden changes in muscle tone, can be a sign of a seizure in a young child. For this reason, the EEG test to look for a seizure focus is a common one in pediatric practice.

The test is done by sticking an array of small round electrodes on the surface of the child's head. The electrodes are placed in a specific order and relationship to one another and then are connected to the EEG machine with a fine wire. Sometimes the electrode array is arranged on the inner surface of a special cap, which the technician then places on the child's head. The test usually takes about a half hour to do. The result looks like a series of parallel wavy lines, which are traditionally recorded on paper but these days are mostly displayed on a computer screen. The results of an EEG are usually not available for several hours at least. The technicians who do them are usually quite good at spotting obvious seizure activity, but the tracing needs to be interpreted by a specialist—a neurologist.

The principal difficulty in getting a good EEG reading on a child is the same as for an MRI scan—often children do not understand or cooperate with what we are doing. The test itself does not hurt at all. The worst complaint one hears about EEG tests is that the jelly the technician uses to secure the electrodes to the child's scalp can be sticky stuff to shampoo out later. However, the child needs to lie quietly enough for the EEG technician to get a good tracing on the machine. In addition, it is often useful to get one

EEG reading while the patient is awake and another while he is asleep. For both these reasons, children are frequently given sedatives to relax them for the EEG. This is entirely safe, as long as the proper precautions are taken for the use of these drugs, primarily monitoring the child's oxygen level.

COMMUNICATION CHECKLIST FOR PARENTS

1. Is the doctor going to order any tests for your child?
2. If yes, which tests, and specifically how will the results help in your child's care?
3. If a blood test is needed, is there time to use EMLA or other pain-killing cream?
4. If a blood test is needed, and the doctor also plans to order an intravenous line, can the blood be drawn through the fresh intravenous line? (This saves the child an additional needle stick.)
5. Will the doctor share the specific test results with you?
6. If your child needs an X-ray or scan, will the doctor show you the images and point out any abnormalities on them?
7. If your child is being seen by someone other than his or her regular doctor, how will the test results be communicated to your child's regular doctor?

Chapter 5

PUTTING IT ALL TOGETHER

THE DIFFERENTIAL DIAGNOSIS

T he last three chapters have led you through the three components of the diagnostic triad—medical history, physical examination, and laboratory tests. Now you will learn about the step in the process that involves all three components—how doctors use the components to solve the puzzle of a child's illness. Sometimes this is a simple process, sometimes not. On some occasions just one of the three components predominate in the solution, other times all three are needed equally. No matter which component is most important in a particular situation, your child's doctor reaches an answer using a checklist called the *differential diagnosis*. A parent who wants to understand how doctors solve medical mysteries must understand how we use this important mental tool.

The differential diagnosis is a list of diagnoses, ordered from most likely to least likely, which could best explain your child's chief complaint. In the more simple cases, the doctor has an informal, mental checklist; in more complicated situations, she writes the list down in the record. This written menu of possibilities then serves as a guide for how to proceed.

Ideally, the best diagnosis is one that would be consistent with all aspects of your child's medical history, physical examination, and laboratory results. If more than one diagnosis could fit, then the goal is to eliminate possibilities from the list. This may require nothing more than revisiting the medical history with some additional questions or rechecking something on the physical examination. If after performing these tasks there are still possibilities on the differential diagnosis list, then additional tests may be needed to solve the puzzle. Very complicated cases may require the opinion of one or more subspecialist physicians (more about this in chapter 8), especially if the differential diagnosis list contains possibilities with serious implications, such as disorders requiring complicated therapies. The medical chart then becomes a way for the experts to record their own lists and comment upon those of their colleagues.

For common chief complaints, though, the differential diagnosis list is quite standard, and doctors are taught to evaluate children with these problems by working down the standard list. This chapter will help parents learn what is generally on this differential diagnosis list for common problems. As we did for the physical examination, we will begin at the top of the body and work our way down. Some of this will already sound familiar to you from earlier chapters but this chapter will put matters in a new light by showing you how doctors integrate the history, physical examination, and laboratory results into a conclusion about what is wrong with your child. You will understand that this decision is based upon both significant positive findings—what *is* there, and key negative findings—what is *not* there.

My goal in this chapter, as in the entire book, is not to provide an exhaustive, do-it-yourself resource text with which you can diagnose what is wrong with your child. It is far from that, and that would be a dangerous thing for any parent to do anyway. Rather, this chapter uses a selected list of common childhood complaints to show you how the process of medical reasoning happens, how sometimes the history is paramount, other times the physical examination, and still other times laboratory tests matter most. It is only in working through the differential diagnosis that one can see the interplay of all three. This chapter is about what is going through the doctor's mind and why.

HEADACHE

Headache is a common complaint among children. A good history is the cornerstone of the evaluation of a headache patient, because unless the child is having a severe headache at the time of the exam, there are rarely any positive findings. In some situations, laboratory tests, particularly head CT scans and spinal taps, are important, but usually the history is the key. Of particular importance is if the headache is sudden and new, or an exacerbation of a long-standing symptom.

The differential diagnosis list for a child with headaches contains four main causes, or possibilities: tension, or muscular headache; migraine, or vascular headache; increased pressure inside the skull, such as from a tumor; or referred pain, which means pain that originates from somewhere else. Nearly all children with headache have one of the first two possibilities.

The skull is covered by several layers of muscles. *Tension headache*, the most common cause on the list, represents spasm of these muscles. The identifying factors are that the pain is relatively constant and that it feels like a tight, constricting band around the head. Nausea and vomiting are rarely present. Not surprisingly, tension headache often comes when the child is overtired or stressed in some way. Tension headaches usually come on as the day progresses; the child does not have them first thing in the morning, and they never awaken the child from sleep.

Children with vascular headache, or *migraine*, have quite different symptoms. Vascular headache is characteristically a throbbing pain; to the migraine sufferer, it feels as if there is someone pounding a hammer inside his head. Nausea and vomiting are extremely common with vascular headaches, as is a history of lights or sounds making the pain worse. There is very often a family history for migraine. Parents often notice things that trigger the headaches, such as certain activities or foods.

So-called classical migraine headache involves what is called an *aura*, some characteristic sensation like numbness or seeing flashing lights, which varies with the individual and serves as a warning that a headache is about to start, usually within an hour. A history of an aura is helpful if present, but more commonly the headache just comes on without any such warning.

It is the third item on the list, the possibility that a headache heralds something serious like a brain tumor or infection, that often worries parents the most. Physicians share this worry, even though this cause is very uncommon. As a practical matter, a physician evaluating a child for headache seeks an answer to a key question: does the child need any tests to rule out these serious possibilities?

If the child has other findings that suggest the possibility of an infection, especially fever and a stiff neck, then the spinal tap is important. There are a few aspects of the history that suggest a serious cause like a tumor. Headaches of this sort typically come on gradually, over days or even weeks, with steady worsening of the symptoms. They are frequently worse at night or first thing in the morning, and may awaken a child from sleep. A child may have associated neurological symptoms like numbness and tingling in a hand or difficulty with balance. If any of these things are present, your child's doctor will almost always order a head CT scan because, even if it does not show a cause for the headache, a normal CT is very reassuring to both the doctor and the parents.

Finally, headache can also be caused by pain referred from a nearby part of the body, such as the middle ear or the sinuses. Systemic illness of many sorts may come with a headache.

The doctor uses the physical examination to decide about these possibilities.

EAR PROBLEMS

Earaches are an extremely common pediatric complaint. They are so common that a doctor seeing a toddler for fever will put ear infection high on the differential diagnosis list even if no signs suggestive of it, such as pulling or tugging at the ears, is provided by the parent in the history. In a busy outpatient clinic, it can seem as if the doctor assumes every young patient with fever has otitis media until proven otherwise. As you learned in the last chapter, middle ear infection is painful unless the ear drum ruptures—that often relieves the pressure and the pain with it. Infection in the ear canal causes drainage from the ear and usually pain when the ear is wiggled, although usually not much pain otherwise. Simple fluid in the middle ear, serous otitis, rarely hurts and does not cause fever. Ultimately the history and laboratory tests matter little in diagnosing ear infection; the examination is the gold standard.

Other ear disorders, particularly of the inner ear, can manifest themselves as balance problems, ringing in the ears, or decreased hearing. Sometimes a child's teacher is the first to notice decreased hearing, and we need to consider it on our differential diagnosis list as a possible cause for worsening school performance. In very small children, an important clue to poor hearing is delayed speech development, since children learn to speak by listening to others speak.

We now have the technology to check hearing in very small children, and it is now the standard for all infants to have a hearing screen done shortly after they are born. This is important because early intervention in hearing-impaired children prevents many of the later problems in language development.

EYE PROBLEMS

Diagnosis of children's eye complaints usually requires a combination of the history and the physical examination. Common eye complaints include pain, swelling, drainage from the eye, and non-fused gaze—one eye looks one way and the other eye another. Sometimes an older child will say he has difficulty seeing, or his teacher will question if he sees normally.

A common cause for pain, especially if it is very sharp and quite severe, is a scratch on the cornea, the surface of the eye. This can be a difficult diagnosis to make in preverbal children, especially babies, so doctors need to be alert for it. Such *corneal abrasions* are always on the differential diagnosis list for a baby who is acutely and mysteriously in pain from something. The best way to determine if there is a corneal scratch is to put a drop of fluorescent dye in the eye and then shine an ultraviolet "black light" on the eye; the scratch or abrasion will catch the dye and be obvious. Corneal abrasions hurt but also heal quickly. Eye pain can also come from something in the eye, such as grit or a wayward eyelash. Usually the doctor can see those things easily, and there is usually excessive tearing present as well.

Swelling around the eye can be from infection, especially if the child has fever or eye drainage. Allergies or a reaction to something in the child's environment frequently cause puffy, swollen eyes. Discoloration under the eye, "dark circles," are characteristic of this.

Drainage from the eye, especially if there is also a scratchy feeling in the eye, is often from infection, termed *conjunctivitis*, or "pinkeye" to most people. The conjunctivae are the surfaces the doctor looks at by pulling the lower lid down or the upper lid up; they are bright red in children with conjunctivitis, and the whole surface of the eye is often pink or red with inflammation. The infection may be in one eye or in both. Chronically red, itchy eyes with drainage but with less inflammation of the conjunctivae are often caused by allergies.

MOUTH, NOSE, AND THROAT PROBLEMS

As most parents know, the most common complaint arising from this part of a child's anatomy is sore throat. Other common problems include painful sores inside the mouth, runny nose, and nosebleed.

The differential diagnosis for sore throat lists infection at the top—and very little else. The principal issue is not infection itself, but the cause of the infection—respiratory viruses, strep bacteria, and, if the tonsils are quite large, infectious mononucleosis, an infection caused by another virus. Accompanying symptoms help make the distinction: clear drainage from the nose, dry cough, and smaller tonsils makes a viral infection more likely than strep; high fever and large, swollen tonsils with pus on them make strep more likely. However, these tendencies are not clear-cut because the doctor needs a laboratory test—a throat culture—to tell which of these it is. This is an instance where a history and physical examination alone, though helpful, cannot answer a key question.

Painful sores inside the mouth are a common problem in children. Most of the time, they are on the sides of the mouth, but sometimes they extend across the tongue. Herpes virus is a common cause, resulting in a condition called *herpetic stomatitis*.

One of my teachers called this "the worst disease in pediatrics" for the way it can make children miserable with a fever and a mouthful of painful sores. There is a laboratory test for herpes to confirm the diagnosis. Another common cause for painful mouth sores is *aphthous stomatitis*, the common canker sore. These are less severe and, unlike herpes, do not come in crops with fever; their cause is unknown.

Runny noses are ubiquitous in small children, nearly always caused by respiratory viruses. There are other possibilities, however, chiefly allergies, and both conditions deserve a place on the differential diagnosis list for *rhinorrhea*, physician's fancy name for runny nose. The important distinction is found in the history, in the association with other symptoms. Allergic runny noses are more chronic, may come with other common allergic symptoms such as itching eyes, and do not come with infectious symptoms like fever. Respiratory viral infection often causes fever, cough, sore throat, and general malaise.

Another common childhood nose ailment is frequent bloody noses, something known as *epistaxis*. This is common during times of the year when the air is dry. The differential diagnosis list for this is short: normal child, a child with an abnormality such as a single blood vessel near the surface and prone to bleed, or a child with some underlying bleeding problem. Most children are in the first group. The history usually is key, particularly the severity and frequency of the bleeding. Whereas most normal children will have nosebleeds from time to time, severe bleeding always from the same spot suggests the second possibility, and severe bleeding from several places in both nostrils suggests the third. Testing a child's blood is sometimes needed to identify those with underlying bleeding problems. As you would expect, however, those children will usually have a history of bleeding from other places besides the nose; for example, they might bruise easily.

LUNG PROBLEMS

Chief complaints involving the lungs are among the most common reasons for a parent to bring their child to the doctor, so any physician who cares for children ought to be quite skilled in figuring them out. The principal ones are difficulty breathing and cough. The differential diagnosis of lung problems is a challenging one, but it is also one containing all three legs of the diagnostic triad in roughly equivalent degrees of importance.

Functionally, children's lung complaints are divided between infectious and noninfectious causes—pneumonia or something else, and, if pneumonia, from what? Wheezing, often from asthma, is the most common noninfectious cause of respiratory distress. (Asthma has undergone some tinkering with its name, being sometimes called *reactive airways disease*.) The differential list is complicated, though, by the existence of conditions that encompass both infectious and noninfectious causes. For example, some viral infections are notorious for causing wheezing. One of these is *bronchiolitis*, a lung infection common in children under six months of age. Viral infection is also a common trigger for wheezing in children who already have underlying asthma. So it is a complicated issue. The practical result of the diagnostic overlap of many lung complaints is that your child's doctor may not be able to tell what the cause is, requiring him to treat several possibilities and see what happens.

Cough is another symptom with a difficult-to-sort-out differential diagnosis list. The doctor is often guided by what else the child has. For example, the cough of bacterial pneumonia often brings up lots of mucus from the child's chest, whereas the cough of viral infection and asthma is usually dry. Chronic sinus drainage, from infection or allergies, also causes cough.

An experienced physician uses his stethoscope to help decide what the lung problem is: asthma causes wheezing, sometimes with a few crackles, whereas pneumonia causes crackles and often decreased breath sounds over part of the lungs. The chest X-ray is usually helpful in sorting these possibilities, so a doctor examining a child with breathing troubles is usually asking himself: does the child need an X-ray?

HEART PROBLEMS

Disorders of the heart are generally more difficult to diagnose than the disorders we have discussed thus far in the chapter. The child's history can be suggestive of heart problems. For example, the child may tire easily and have looked occasionally dusky to the parents, usually over a period of weeks to months. Older children sometimes can tell you they have felt odd flutterings in their pulse.

Pediatric heart disease is different from adult heart disease in that the majority of affected children will have been born with a malformed heart. It is very unusual for such children to have escaped diagnosis once they are a few years old. Nearly all major forms of congenital heart disease get diagnosed long before that, usually in infancy. Children can, however, get several different kinds of acquired heart disease. Therefore the key issue in the history is whether the child was previously normal and then got sick or has always been ill in some way.

Although the history is helpful for diagnosing heart disease, as with the lungs, it is the physical examination that tells the doctor the most about the heart and blood vessels. One laboratory test, the echocardiogram, has emerged as by far the easiest and most important way to identify what is wrong. Even so, it is the doctor with a stethoscope who decides that an echocardiogram is needed; the physical examination is still key to that decision.

ABDOMINAL PROBLEMS

Abdominal complaints—pain, vomiting, and diarrhea—account for a large number of children's visits to the doctor. For these children, the medical history is preeminent in the assessment. If you bring your child in with such symptoms, you can expect the doctor to spend quite a bit of time on the history. She will often ask you similar questions various ways in an effort to zero in on the exact sequence of events.

The differential diagnosis list for abdominal problems is a very long one, perhaps the longest in pediatric practice. The first fork in the road in evaluating this complaint is timing; the doctor needs to decide if the problem is acute, meaning of recent onset, or chronic, meaning having been present for days, weeks, or even years. If it has been a chronic problem, the doctor will need to know if the problem is constant or intermittent. If it is the latter, the precise timing of when it gets better or worse, and what other things are associated with this waxing and waning, is key.

If the problem is chronic, the doctor is often unable to arrive at a diagnosis without various laboratory tests and several visits with you and your child to go over the results. It is not a good idea to bring your child to an acute-care, walk-in facility for complaints of this sort; it is far better to see a doctor in a situation that allows for a more thorough evaluation, such as an office appointment. If you take your child to the emergency department to discover a cause for long-standing symptoms, you are very likely going to be disappointed.

Chronic abdominal pain is a very common pediatric ailment, so all pediatricians and experienced family doctors are well trained to evaluate it. The history is paramount. Initially the doctor sorts the complaint into one of two categories: organic or functional. As you read in chapter 2, these terms, although useful, are also laden with implications that can cloud your child's evaluation.

There are several items on the doctor's differential diagnosis list for chronic abdominal pain, but functional abdominal pain, discomfort for which the doctor cannot find any physical cause, is extremely common in children. It probably accounts for the majority of children with mild to moderate intermittent pain. Every parent has heard their child complain from time to time that "my tummy hurts." As with tension headaches in adults, abdominal pain seems to express for children's bodies some dissatisfaction with current circumstances. The hallmarks of functional abdominal pain are that it is associated with specific times, such as Monday morning before school or before a weekly piano lesson, and that it is not severe or debilitating. Important, too, is that there are no serious systemic findings like fever.

There are several items on the differential diagnosis list for chronic abdominal pain that are organic, not functional. One is chronic constipation, something diagnosed by the history, although often the doctor also uses the physical examination because he can feel hard stool in the child's lower intestines when he pushes on the lower left part of the abdomen. An abdominal X-ray is also helpful in this situation. Ulcers sometimes occur in children, and the symptoms are typically those of chronic pain. Often a parent will give a child complaining of stomach pain an over-the-counter antacid; a significant point in the history is whether anything helped the pain, and antacids usually give temporary relief.

Another uncommon, but not rare, condition that manifests itself as chronic pain is called *Meckel's diverticulum*. This is a congenital problem in which an abnormal bit of stomach tissue appears lower down in the intestines, where it secretes stomach acid just as normal stomach tissue does. But whereas the stomach's lining protects it from the acid, the intestines have no such protection, and so the Meckel's causes pain and often bleeding into the stools. It is diagnosed with a special laboratory scan and needs surgery to fix.

There are several kinds of chronic intestinal inflammations that, although uncommon, are serious diseases if present. Two of them, *Crohn's disease* and *ulcerative colitis*, are possibilities your child's doctor may consider. Both nearly always have other associated findings with the pain, such as fevers, weight loss (or failure to grow normally), and diarrhea, often with blood in it. Both have laboratory tests that are essential for making the diagnosis. If either of these conditions are high on the doctor's differential diagnosis list, he will order these tests for your child.

Acute abdominal pain is an entirely different matter from chronic pain, especially if it is severe; acute, severe pain needs prompt attention. A variant of this situation would be a severe exacerbation of chronic pain; this should not wait for medical evaluation, either. As you read in the section about abdominal examination technique, when a doctor evaluates a child with acute abdominal pain, he is looking first to answer a simple question: does this child need to see a surgeon now?

If the answer is yes, then of course the doctor will call the surgeon, sometimes without ordering any tests at all. If the answer is clearly no, then she can proceed with the child's evaluation. Sometimes the answer is maybe, in which case she will often order some X-rays, an ultrasound, or blood tests and decide from these results whether to call the surgeon.

Acute abdominal pain often needs time to reveal its cause, so waiting for some tests, then reexamining the child later, is a very useful way to proceed. Impatient, even frustrated parents should understand that diagnosing what is wrong is often difficult. Observation of the child with several repeat examinations to see if anything has changed is a standard, logical way to handle the symptom. Sometimes this process takes hours, and there is nothing we can or should do to rush things because answering the surgical question— yes or no—is crucial to giving your child the best care. In situations like this, the child may be admitted to the hospital to allow such serial examinations every few hours. Then if your child needs surgery, he is already in the right place to have it.

You read in chapter 3 about what doctors look for in those repeated examinations on a child we suspect has what we term a *surgical abdomen*, meaning a child who might need an abdominal operation. The most typical characteristic is rebound tenderness; it nearly always indicates a need for an operation. Other kinds of abdominal pain are also characteristic of different disorders. Depending upon the history, the exact kind of pain determines what items are near the top of the differential diagnosis list. For example, the nerves inside the intestine are particularly sensitive to stretching. Blocked intestines get stretched, and the pain from this stretching occurs in a particular way. This pain comes in waves, being present for several minutes and then subsiding for several minutes, so-called *colicky* pain. In contrast, pain from an inflamed liver (*hepatitis*) or an inflamed pancreas (*pancreatitis*), an organ at the back of the abdominal area, is a steady, unremitting pain. Pancreatitis is notorious for causing a restless kind of pain because there is no position the person can assume that will make it better. Both hepatitis and pancreatitis are diagnosed by blood tests and often ultrasound scans.

Vomiting is another common chief complaint among children. Beyond the frequency of it, vomiting is important primarily for what it contains. Fresh blood indicates bleeding, of course, which may be coming either from the stomach or the lower part of the *esophagus*, the swallowing tube to the stomach. The presence of greenish-yellow bile in the emesis (vomit) tells the doctor the intestines are backing up, which is probably why the child is vomiting. Blood that has been in the stomach for a few hours is no longer red; it turns black from the action of stomach acid and looks like coffee grounds. Unless the doctor actually sees your child vomit any of these things, it is the history you provide that will affect what ailments are on the doctor's differential diagnosis list.

The most common cause for vomiting is infection, usually from a virus—the common "stomach flu," or what a doctor calls *gastroenteritis*. (You can see medical jargon at work here; this impressive term is nothing more than a stringing together of the Latin root words for stomach, intestines, and inflammation.) Often the child will have some diarrhea, abdominal pain, and fever as well. This diagnosis is made almost exclusively by the history and physical examination because there are no specific physical examination findings or laboratory tests.

One of the serious causes of vomiting is blockage of the intestinal tract. As you would expect, this kind of vomiting is usually severe and constant, although there are a few conditions that cause only intermittent obstruction, and therefore only intermittent symptoms. If the doctor suspects such a blockage, he will order X-rays to diagnosis it, often barium studies or CT scans. Sometimes the intestines are not blocked but just behave as if they are. Such a shutting down of the normal transit of intestinal contents is called an *ileus*. It is diagnosed by X-ray.

Abnormal stooling is a common reason for parents to bring their child to the doctor, especially if it occurs among infants and toddlers. Diarrhea is the most frequent complaint, although this word means different things to different people. One parent's definition of diarrhea is another's version of normal. A doctor's definition varies with the age of the child; babies often have a stool after each feeding, less as they get older, but even an infant's stools should not be liquid. In general, diarrhea means liquid stools occurring more frequently than normal for your child.

The complaint can have several causes, and your history will be crucial in helping the doctor arrange the list of which possibilities are most likely. Overall, though, infection is by far the most common. Diarrhea from ordinary viral gastroenteritis often comes with mild to moderate abdominal pain and fever. More severe intestinal infection often results in pain of the waxing and waning, cramping variety. The worst infections cause bloody stools and have high fevers; these are often caused by bacteria. If your child's doctor suspects one of these, he can test the stools for them.

All forms of diarrhea can result in dehydration from fluid lost in the stools, particularly in infants. The doctor identifies dehydration with a combination of the history (decreased urination), the physical examination (fast heart rate, a sunken fontanel, dry mouth, or abnormally doughy skin) and laboratory tests (chemistry group and urinalysis).

Sometimes parents bring their child to the doctor not for diarrhea or constipation but for abnormal stools themselves. It is never normal for a child to have blood in the stool. Blood from the lower end of the intestinal tract—the large intestines and rectum—looks red. In contrast, bleeding from upstream in the intestinal tract—the stomach—causes black stools like sticky tar from the action of the child's digestive tract on the blood. The intestinal tract is long, and the source of bleeding can be hard to locate. Usually it requires special tests, one of which calls for a specialist to look inside the child's upper or lower intestinal tract with a long, flexible lighted tube called an *endoscope* to see where the blood is coming from directly.

One final stool problem doctors encounter is abnormally colored stools. One common pediatric patient is the child with reddish stools whose parent is concerned is bleeding. There is a fast and easy test we can do on stool to see if this reddish color is caused by blood. Generally, however, funny-colored stools reflect something unusual the child ate or drank. One exception to this are stools that are abnormally clay-colored; this reflects the absence of normal bile in the stool, and it is an observation with potentially serious implications because it indicates some problem in the liver.

As you can see, diagnosing a child's abdominal complaints can be quite challenging. The possible items on the differential diagnosis list are many, and several of them are quite serious. Abdominal problems, more than most other aspects of diagnostic detective work, require contributions from all three legs of the diagnostic triad of history, physical examination, and laboratory testing. Informed parents can be extraordinarily helpful to their child's doctor in solving this puzzle.

URINARY PROBLEMS

Evaluation of children's urinary tract problems leans more heavily on the laboratory testing aspect than on the physical examination and the history, although the last of these has a role to play. Compared with abdominal pain, the differential diagnosis list for urinary complaints is much shorter and less complicated. Typical urinary symptoms are pain with urination, blood in the urine, too frequent urination, or what doctors call *urgency*, which is the sensation of a sudden and immediate need to urinate. Toilet-trained children may show their distress by wetting themselves.

Near the top of any differential diagnosis list for urinary tract complaints is infection, so a urine culture and urinalysis is usually the key test. Infants and young toddlers with a urinary tract infection may not have these typical symptoms but instead will have abdominal pain and fever. This is why you will see doctors order urine cultures on children who have vague pains but no specific urinary complaints. We nearly always get a urine culture on an infant or toddler with a fever if we cannot find some obvious explanation for the high temperature, such as an infected ear, throat, or lung.

Abnormally colored urine is another reason parents bring children to the doctor. Most parents know that urine color is generally related to its concentration; well-hydrated children have more frequent passage of clear, dilute urine, whereas dehydrated children urinate less frequently and their urine is darker-colored. Sometimes, however, urine can have abnormal color. Red or pink urine often indicates fresh blood, which is never normal, and brown or cola-colored urine can mean problems in the liver or the kidney. All of these things are easy to tell with the simple urinalysis test.

Children who have urinary tract infections often need tests to make sure they have no problems with their urinary tracts. We have several useful tests for looking at the structure of the kidneys and bladder, as well as the *ureter*, the tube connecting the two. The most common of these is the ultrasound scan. It gives a painless, risk-free assessment of the kidneys. This scan is the easiest way to tell if there is any blockage of urine flow from the child's kidneys down to the bladder. If the ultrasound does not give the information we need, X-ray tests with contrast provide a detailed image of these organs.

EXTREMITIES

The most common complaints in this region are pain and swelling, the differential diagnosis of which derives mostly from the physical examination and X-rays. Some points of the history are important, however. For example, the doctor will ask the obvious question of whether there was a history of injury to the arm or leg. He will also ask how long the pain has been there. Pain from injury should have a sudden onset.

The hallmarks of a broken bone are pain, swelling, and deformity. Children frequently get so-called green stick fractures, in which the bone has its surface stretched and cracked but not broken through. This results in a nondisplaced fracture, one in which the ends of the bones are still aligned with each other. Fractures are simple to diagnose; expect the doctor to X-ray any arm or leg that is swollen and painful.

The history is particularly important for children with one or more swollen, tender joints, or *arthritis*. Although this word is commonly used by nonphysicians, when a doctor says *arthritis*, he means that the joint has more than just pain—it also has the typical signs of inflammation of redness, increased warmth, swelling, and tenderness to touch. Often a young child with an arthritic joint will not complain about it but will instead just quit using it; parents will note that the child refuses to use an arm or to bear weight on one leg. Arthritis in the hip can be particularly difficult to localize in a child; for example, a child with hip inflammation will sometimes complain of pain in the knee.

The differential diagnosis for arthritis, if it is not the result of an injury like a twisted ankle or knee, is much more complicated than the list of possible causes for extremity swelling and pain between joints. For the latter, usually an X-ray will give the answer to the question: is the bone broken or not? In contrast, arthritis has many potential causes, from infection to obscure systemic diseases. Doctors usually begin a swollen joint evaluation with an X-ray just to be sure no bone is broken, but if it is not, we frequently need a battery of blood tests and special scans to decide what could be wrong.

SKIN PROBLEMS

Any crowded waiting room in a pediatric clinic or emergency department will have at least a few children waiting to see the doctor for a rash. As you read previously, diagnosis of skin problems is primarily a matter of pattern recognition, which is an aspect of the physical examination. The history can also be helpful, particularly when a parent can tell you precisely when the rash began, how it moved over the body, and what else, if anything, was associated with the appearance of the rash. In spite of those important issues in the history, diagnosis of rashes is well known to be something that can be done by a skilled examiner from photographs of patients for whom she has no history at all.

It is fair to ask what the importance is of even knowing what caused a rash, particularly those causing no symptoms. Many rashes, perhaps the majority of them, come and go without us being able to tell what caused them; the skin is a sensitive organ and reacts to many things in the environment. Babies especially have sensitive skin. One thing the examiner is looking for is evidence that the rash is part of a serious, underlying disorder in the child. If it does appear to be part of a larger problem, then the differential diagnosis list becomes very long indeed, and some of the diseases on that list are serious ones. If that is not the case, then the possibilities narrow considerably. Thus from the doctor's perspective, rashes usually are minor problems, but every once in a while their implications are huge. Even if the doctor has no idea what caused a rash, she nearly always can do things to relieve the symptoms, such as prescribe anti-itching medications.

NEUROLOGICAL PROBLEMS

The differential diagnosis list for neurological problems is a long one, and choosing between the items often takes specialized skills. Moreover, unlike the case with rashes, the implications for the child with neurological problems are often quite significant. This is why a child with neurological complaints like weakness, poor coordination, altered state of consciousness, unusual sensations, or seizures will often need to be evaluated by a specialist—a neurologist.

Even though the differential diagnosis list for neurological problems is long, and many of the things on it are uncommon, rare, or even esoteric, key points of the medical history help to separate the possibilities. Of particular importance are the timing of onset and progression. For example, has the child had the problem for hours, days, weeks, months, or always? Is it progressively worse, never relenting, does it wax and wane, or has it been the same for a long time? Also important is whether the symptom, such as weakness, affects the child's entire body or just parts of it.

Significant neurological complaints in children include the obvious ones of numbness and weakness in an arm or a leg. Poor balance, ringing in the ears, and headache are other examples. For young children, especially toddlers, what we call *developmental milestones* are important; delays in holding up the head, rolling over, talking, walking, and interpersonal development can all be signs of neurological problems. This is one reason your child's doctor assesses these things at well-child visits—to identify children who could have a neurological disorder.

The practical decision for a pediatrician examining a child with symptoms of potential neurological origin is whether that child should see a neurologist, and if so, when. Pediatricians are familiar with many of the disorders on the neurological differential diagnosis list, but there are many disorders that are unusual, or even rare. Many neurological conditions of childhood appear slowly and are not immediately dangerous. For that reason a pediatrician evaluating a child in this situation is usually trying to decide if there is anything that needs immediate action or any tests that need to be done immediately. If not, then a referral to a neurologist is often the best way to proceed.

One possible neurological problem frequently on the differential diagnosis list is seizures. You read in chapter 4 about tests we use to determine if a child has seizures. For an evaluating doctor going down his list of possible diagnoses, the practical question is if the child has anything in the history to suggest seizures; if so, then an EEG is usually indicated.

Seizures in children, especially very young children and infants, can be very difficult, even impossible to identify just by looking at the child. All manner of spells—limpness, staring, funny twitches, altered awareness, and more—can be attributable to seizures, and the spells can last only seconds. After a seizure is over, it often takes some time for a child to appear and act completely normal, so if your child is seeing the doctor for any mysterious spells that could be seizures, be ready for questions about precisely what happened after the spell stopped.

ɤ   ɤ   ɤ

In sum, the differential diagnosis is like a running mental commentary doctors carry on in their minds. This internal dialogue begins with the opening of the medical history interview, moves through the physical examination, and does not pause even once we have received back the last test result from the laboratory or radiology department. The process continues; we often learn additional things to ponder from further conversation with the parents or a recheck of the physical examination.

Medicine is not really a science. It is an art, although one guided by science. The most artful doctors are those who can maintain a balance between using what they already know to direct what they need to do, such as tests, and remaining open to modifying what they do based upon new information, such as a new symptom the child develops during the evaluation. These doctors also learn to cultivate and ultimately trust their own intuition. The best doctors, of course, are those who also are good communicators with parents and children, who explain what they are doing and why.

What follows next is an example of a patient for whom the differential diagnosis changed several times in crucial ways. The child's problem was at first obscure and not even on the doctor's initial differential diagnosis list. As the story evolved, however, the doctor kept revising his mental list, testing new hypotheses about what was wrong, and ultimately arriving at the right answer. Like some of our previous vignettes, this one is a made-up pastiche. But also like the previous ones, it is based on true stories I have heard over the years.

The story's purpose is to illustrate how a parent who understands how doctors think can streamline and facilitate their child's care. Beyond that, insightful parents can do more than facilitate—they can have a major positive influence on what happens to their child. The story begins when the doctor picks up the chart from the rack by the examination room door and walks into the room where a mother waits with her three-year-old son.

"The nurse tells me young Ryan here has had belly pain and been vomiting. What can you tell me about that?"

"It first started a week ago yesterday, quite suddenly. He was completely fine before that. He's had some occasional vomiting in the past, with the flu, but nothing like this."

"How is this different?"

"He seems just fine for several hours, even as long as a day, then seems to develop stomach pains—it makes him stop what he's doing, and sometimes it makes him cry out. He then lies on the floor and curls into a little ball. Then, after a few minutes he seems better, then worse again. Each episode comes completely out of the blue, lasts an hour or so, and usually ends with vomiting. Then he's fine—no fever, normal appetite, normal activities—until the next bout."

"What's the longest he's gone without an episode?"

"About eighteen hours. At least one of them woke him up from a sound sleep."

"Has he had anything else with this, been sick in any way?"

"Nothing that I can say. He's been eating the same things in between these spells, hasn't had any fever, rash, or diarrhea. He is having regular bowel movements, at least once each day, and they've seemed like his usual—formed, not loose. The reason I brought him in now is that he's had four of these spells in the last twelve hours, hasn't wanted to eat anything, and the pain during each spell seems to be getting worse."

"What does it look like when he vomits?"

"A few times it's been what he's eaten, but most of the time it just looks like greenish mucous—no blood or anything."

This brief exchange accomplished several very important things. The mother told the doctor exactly why she was there at that particular time and she clearly described her son's symptoms— what they were, what they were associated with, whether there were any aggravating or alleviating factors, if he ever had any similar symptoms before. She also noticed what we call key negatives, things that are significant for their absence, such as fever, rash, and change in bowel habits.

Already the doctor is building in his mind a differential diagnosis list. This child's problem appeared to be a noninfectious one. Even though viral gastroenteritis is by far the most common cause of this complaint, in this child the vomiting was present for some time, longer than typical for infection, and there was nothing else that fit with that diagnosis, such as fever, rash, and malaise. The doctor is probably thinking along the lines of diagnoses that involve obstruction of the intestinal tract. This is suggested by the colicky nature of the pain and the bile in the emesis. The obstruction needed to be intermittent, though, since in between episodes the child seems fine.

There is a principle of medical diagnosis, one that you will read more about in the next chapter, that "common things are common." This means we should put near the top of our differential diagnosis list things that are common, even though everything in the story might not fit with that common item. The doctor in this story is doing just that; whereas bowel obstruction is rare, constipation is extremely common, especially in recently toilet-trained toddlers who do not like to stop what they are doing to go to the bathroom. Constipation can cause pain, and perhaps the vomiting was from some other cause. So even though this mother said her son's bowel movements were "normal," the doctor appropriately revisits that issue.

"You said Ryan's bowel movements have been normal. Are they hard or soft? Are you sure there's been no diarrhea?"

"I've not noticed any change, and he's never been constipated."

We will skip over the past medical, social, and family histories, as well as the systems review because they give the doctor no new important information in this particular case. The doctor proceeds to the physical examination with a differential diagnosis list that contains a series of things that can cause intermittent and partial intestinal obstruction in an otherwise normal child.

The child's physical examination is entirely normal until the doctor reaches the abdominal portion. Particularly important are the key negatives; the child is well grown, well nourished, and has normal vital signs. As the doctor feels the child's abdomen he wonders if he senses a fullness on the left side of the belly. It is not firm, so it is not stool in the lower intestines (which, if present, would suggest constipation in spite of what the mother said). It is not particularly tender, so it is not some inflammatory mass like an infected abscess. It is so vague the doctor goes back to feel it again a few minutes later after he completes the rest of the examination; now he is unsure if he feels anything at all.

The doctor decides to order an abdominal X-ray, plus a CBC. The former is an excellent screening test for blockage of the intestines or ileus, and also for a lower intestine filled with constipated stool; the latter is a way to see if the child has suffered occult bleeding into the intestine. As the child goes off to the radiology department, the doctor moves on to evaluate another child in the interim.

When the child returns from radiology, the doctor goes to see him again. In his mind, he still has chronic constipation at the top of his differential diagnosis list, simply because it is so common as a cause of intermittent abdominal pain in toddlers. He is even thinking about acting on that presumption by ordering an enema for the child.

The mother tells him she thinks another pain episode is coming on. Indeed, the child is curled up in a ball on the stretcher and complaining that his "tummy hurts." The doctor uncurls the child and discovers that now his abdomen seems more tender, although there are no signs of a surgical situation such as rebound. The doctor senses again that there may be something unusual on the left side of the child's abdomen. So instead of ordering an enema, he orders an abdominal ultrasound.

The ultrasound shows what looks to be a fluid-filled mass about the size of a lemon where the doctor had been feeling. The results of the abdominal X-ray suggest that something is partially obstructing the child's small intestine. The doctor then calls a pediatric surgeon to evaluate the child, who agrees that there is something in the intestine that should not be there, and orders a CT scan, the definitive test to define what the unusual something is. The CT shows a duplication cyst, an abnormal congenital blind pouch of the intestine that had not caused the child any trouble until now. The surgeon operates on the child, removes the cyst, and the child recovers uneventfully.

This made-up vignette is true-to-life in the way it shows how the diagnostic process works. When it works well, it is a partnership between the doctor and the parent, as illustrated here. The result is an expeditious evaluation, a satisfied parent, and a child who gets the right tests and the right treatment. Often the diagnosis is simple and obvious; sometimes it is not. Either way, it is entirely appropriate for you to ask your child's doctor about what his differential diagnosis list is for your child's ailment. Good doctors, no matter how busy, welcome even a brief opportunity to explain what they are doing to a receptive parent, especially one who is savvy enough about how medicine actually is practiced to understand what we are saying and why.

Now that we have a diagnosis, our next chapter is about treatment. You will learn about the kinds of therapies doctors can offer your child, how we think about them, and how we choose between them.

COMMUNICATION CHECKLIST FOR PARENTS

1. When you have finished your history-taking conversation with the doctor, ask what she is thinking about as possible causes; make sure in your own mind you have told her everything relevant you can think of about those possibilities.
2. If, at the end of her physical examination, the doctor is unsure of the diagnosis, ask her what is on her list of possibilities and how she will choose among them.
3. If the doctor recommends tests, ask how they will help her distinguish among the items on the list.
4. If the doctor changes her mind, ask her what led her to do so.

Chapter 6

WHAT TO DO

How Doctors Choose Therapies for Your Child

You have read in the previous chapters how a physician uses the history, the physical examination, and laboratory tests to formulate a differential diagnosis and then decide what your child's problem is. That is all well and good, and it is very useful information for parents to have so they can understand how doctors reach decisions, but the key question most parents have is this: now that the doctor knows what is wrong, what is he going to do about it? Parents tend to think of therapies, particularly how to use prescription medications, differently than physicians do. This chapter will give you a doctor's perspective and will help you understand why doctors do things that can seem mysterious to parents.

How doctors decide what to do with a child who has a particular problem is one issue, but there is an important related question: what do we do if we are not sure, or if we have little idea what is wrong? Parents may find this last possibility disconcerting, but in fact varieties of this dilemma occur frequently. Diagnostic uncertainty represents a spectrum of doubt. On one end of the continuum, the doctor, although having some reservations, may still be reasonably sure about what a child's problem is and what to do; on the other end, he may be completely mystified and unsure what course of action is best.

Yet even children who are diagnostic enigmas need some kind of therapy, at least temporarily. A child whose head hurts still feels the pain even though the doctor may have no explanation for it; a child with an itchy rash still scratches even though the cause is at first unclear. Thus even though a purist might insist on the logical progression of a child's evaluation—first diagnosis, then therapy—this is not always practical or appropriate. Quite often we doctors are forced to do what we think is best in spite of the uncertainty.

The best way for a parent to think about medical treatments as a doctor thinks about them is to understand the difference between what we call *specific* and *supportive* therapies. The first kind, specific treatment, is easy to understand. Certain kinds of infections provide pure examples of it. For example, when a child has an infection in his bloodstream or his urine, we nearly always can identify exactly which bacteria are causing the infection by growing the microorganisms in the laboratory from a blood culture or a urine culture of the sort you read about in chapter 4. We can then test a panel of antibiotic medications on the bacteria to see which one kills the bacteria with the lowest chance of side effects; the result is specific treatment tailored to the child's specific situation.

Even though treatment of infections is a good example of specific treatment—perhaps the purest one—often even that situation is not clear-cut. This happens, for example, when we are using antibiotics relatively less specifically—when we are sure a child has an infection but we are not sure with what. This is an example of a treatment further down on the spectrum of diagnostic certainty.

Doctors classify some infections as clinical syndromes rather than specific entities caused by specific microorganisms. There are many examples of this: pneumonia (infection of the lungs), and otitis media (infection of the middle ear). We know these are infectious processes, but for one or more reasons we cannot tell what the offending microorganism is.

The principal reason we cannot be sure is that, unlike blood or urinary tract infection, we cannot obtain a sample of the infected material from lungs or ears to test in the laboratory. Blood and urine samples, although they involve the pain of a poke in the arm with a needle or sometimes a catheter into a child's bladder, are relatively easy to get. If bacteria grow from either of these samples, the answer is clear.

Respiratory infections are more complicated to diagnose specifically. Pneumonia often causes a child to cough up phlegm, which, to a doctor and even to a parent, looks infected—it is often discolored, for example. One might think it would be an easy thing to send some of this material to the laboratory to see what bacteria are growing in it, just as we do for blood and urine. It is true that a child's lungs normally have no bacteria in them, so if we do find bacteria, this results in the diagnosis of pneumonia. Unfortunately, coughed-up phlegm always has bacteria in it because it passes through the throat and mouth, which, unlike the lungs, *do* normally have bacteria. We have no practical way to get at what is in the lungs, so we make an educated guess.

Even though we cannot routinely sample what bacteria, if any, are in a child's lungs, special research studies over the years, plus various kinds of indirect information, have given doctors a good idea of the different microorganisms that cause pneumonia. This means when we use a medical history, a physical examination, and laboratory tests (such as a chest X-ray) to determine whether a child has pneumonia, we can make a good guess about the microbial suspects; we then treat according to that guess. Fortunately, most of the time the antibiotics we prescribe for childhood pneumonia cover the most common possibilities. This is not always the case, and sometimes we face some difficult choices about therapy because of it.

A similar situation applies to ear infections. It is possible to diagnose what is causing a child's ear infection by sampling the infected fluid behind the ear drum in the middle ear. It is possible, but not easy, and also not without risk. You read in chapter 4 about the notion of the risk–benefit ratio—the information a test will give is worth the risk of doing the test. We can do a procedure called a *tympanocentesis*, in which we puncture the child's ear drum with a fine needle to get some of the fluid behind it, and we can identify microorganisms in this fluid causing the infection, because the middle ear, like the blood and the urine, is normally completely sterile.

My simply describing tympanocentesis to you should demonstrate why we rarely resort to it; it is uncomfortable and risky because the tiny bones in the middle ear are small and easily damaged. In addition, the procedure requires sedative medications that carry risks of their own. In very unusual instances, we need to do it, but for ordinary ear infections the benefit is not worth the risk. However, research studies on the procedure have told us which microorganisms are the usual offenders, so we make an educated guess based upon those studies.

When a doctor treats your child with antibiotics for either of our two examples—pneumonia or an ear infection—she is using these medications based upon a statistical guess about the most potent drug to use against the bacteria likely to be there. It is a guess that becomes more or less accurate depending upon her experience and skill, but it remains a guess. There is another possibility, actually a common one for both examples; the antibiotics could be totally worthless because the child's ear or lung infection may be caused by a virus. Often we cannot tell which lung and ear infections are caused by viruses. Many are, but children often get antibiotics because we cannot be sure one way or the other.

I have chosen these two examples because they are common ones for children. But there are many others I could have selected, and many that have nothing to do with infections and antibiotics. What all these examples share is the mental balancing the doctor must do, comparing the potential benefit of the treatment with the inherent risk of using it.

Not surprisingly, doctors are much more likely to consider using this kind of "best guess" treatment when the medicine they are considering is safe. This is generally, although not exclusively, true of antibiotics as a group; they are relatively safe. Other medications often have higher risks of side effects. Thus if a doctor is considering a diagnosis for a child that would require treatment with a more toxic drug, she must compare the risk to the child of experiencing one of those side effects to the risk of leaving the condition untreated. Alternatively, she can consider if additional tests, or simply the passage of time, will make a murky diagnostic picture clearer.

Sometimes we extend this way of looking at a child's situation to use an approach we call a *therapeutic trial*. This means we are prescribing a medication just to see if it helps, sometimes even when we are very unsure of the child's diagnosis. For some medications, ones with very specific effects, a therapeutic trial is also referred to as a *diagnostic trial*; in other words, some medications have such well-known and precise effects that determining if a child gets better with them is a way of making a diagnosis—only those patients with a certain condition will respond favorably. Of course, our willingness to use a diagnostic trial approach is very much dictated by how toxic the proposed treatment is; we are only willing to consider a potentially dangerous approach if the condition we are treating is at least as dangerous to the child. The more desperate the situation, the more willing we are to try desperate measures.

This kind of medical treatment is called *empiric*. It is an ancient tradition in medicine, being based upon using what works. Medical empiricism arose from a time when physicians had no knowledge at all about why particular treatments worked; they had theories, nearly all of them fanciful, but no fundamental and correct knowledge. Empiricism was based upon simple observation, and the tradition lives on in many effective folk remedies. Doctors, even modern, high-tech ones, use empiric treatments every day. Sometimes we are reasonably sure of the diagnosis, other times less so.

Specific, diagnosis-guided therapy and empiric, best-guess therapy share the property of treating whatever might be the child's known or presumed medical problem. Sometimes, however, doctors have no treatment at all to cure or even improve the child's condition. Other times, although we have some form of therapy, at the time of the child's evaluation the treatment may seem worse than the condition it treats; perhaps its risk-benefit ratio is highly unfavorable. What do doctors do when we have no specific therapy to offer a child? What we can usually offer is what we call supportive care, something that, like empiricism, is an ancient medical tradition.

Supportive care takes its name from the fact that it is intended to support the ill child—provide comfort, relief of unpleasant symptoms, and needed things like fluids and nutrition—while the child's body heals itself. Put another way, it supports the child's system while the disease or injury, be it a migraine headache, a viral pneumonia, or a sore joint, runs its course. Every parent is familiar with the notion of supportive care, although they may not realize how venerable the practice is. Simple examples include using medications to bring down fever or relieve pain.

Doctors frequently use the concept of supportive care because, at least in pediatrics, the majority of ailments children suffer are self-limited, meaning they will go away on their own without any specific therapy at all. Doctors know this, which is one reason we are judicious in our use of therapeutic trials of medications that could make the situation worse rather than better. Since most things pass, the pediatrician's goal is to relieve the child's uncomfortable symptoms while allowing the problem to pass. We also use therapies to prevent complications of the child's condition, such as using intravenous fluid therapy to keep a vomiting child from becoming dehydrated.

In my experience, some parents are frustrated by the entire notion of supportive care. Such parents have said to me things like: "But doctor, can't you *do* anything?" Their presumption is that, because I cannot give their child a specific remedy, then I am powerless to act, to do anything useful. A few parents even regard situations where we have only supportive care to offer as evidence of modern medicine's failures.

Other parents recognize that supportive care is really an extension of what parents themselves have always done—comforted their child as best they could while the child's malady passes, which it does most of the time. Supportive care has also always been the foundation of medical practice itself, because until only very recently, perhaps fifty years ago or so, doctors had few effective remedies for any disease. Voltaire is credited with the quip that "the art of medicine consists of amusing the patient while nature cures the disease," and until relatively recently, he was correct. So if your child's doctor tells you that there is no specific treatment for what is wrong with your child but still provides you with ways to ease your child's discomfort, it is helpful to remember that you and the doctor are effectively partners in an activity honored by two thousand years of medical practice. I encourage you to approach it not with frustration, but with veneration.

There are a wide variety of supportive therapies doctors prescribe for children. Some of these involve no medications, but many, probably most, include some kind of medicine, so we will examine them first. We will then discuss some common therapies that do not include medications.

The list of medications doctors use gets longer each year. In spite of this enormous variety, there is a core group of medicines that accounts for the great majority of prescriptions written for children. In fact, just two groups of medications, antibiotics and asthma medications, account for about three-quarters of all such prescriptions. The situation with drugs is much like that of laboratory tests. As you read in chapter 4, in spite of the innumerable tests available, doctors evaluating children typically use only a tiny selection most of the time. The same is true of medicines. The standard list of available prescription drugs is the *Physicians' Desk Reference*; it runs to nearly thirty-five hundred pages, yet the list of drugs used for children in the majority of situations would result in a book only a tiny sliver of that size.

What follows are the common categories of those most useful medications—what they are and what the doctor is thinking when she writes a prescription for your child. If you are a parent, you probably already know about many of these medications and have very likely given some of them to your children. Here you will get a view of them through a doctor's eyes, which, I hope, will dispel some of the misconceptions many parents have about how such medications work and when best to use them. My goal, as throughout this book, is to give you the tools to communicate better with your child's doctor by providing you an understanding of the doctor's viewpoint.

ANTIBIOTIC MEDICATIONS

Antibiotics inhibit the growth of bacteria or kill them outright. More than any other drugs, antibiotics symbolize the new power over dis-

WHAT TO DO   159

ease that doctors—particularly doctors who treat children—gained in the middle of the last century. Until about the time of World War II, infections were the leading cause of death in children; after that time the situation changed dramatically. Immunization against common infectious killers, as well as better sanitation, accounted for much of this favorable change, but antibiotics, particularly penicillin, were crucial as well. Children get a lot of infections, typically acute infections, so antibiotics have always been disproportionately important for children compared with adults. They are the largest single category of prescriptions doctors write for children.

There are hundreds of antibiotics available today. This long list is deceptive, though, because virtually all of them belong to a short list of categories. Minor differences between drugs of the same type often do not mean much, and there are sometimes several different brand names for the same drug made by different pharmaceutical companies.

The names for the antibiotics add another layer of confusion, one shared by many other categories of medicines, but which is particularly troublesome for antibiotics because there are so many of them and they are so commonly used in treating children. Medical students dutifully (and painfully) learn what is termed the *generic* name for a drug, a name usually based in some way upon its chemical structure. These generic names, however, are often difficult to remember, pronounce, and spell. The result is that when medical students become doctors, they often use the most common brand name for the drug rather than the generic name; the brand names are shorter and easier to remember because, being devised by pharmaceutical company marketing departments, they were designed that way. Doctors write prescriptions using either brand names or generic names, although usually the pharmacist filling the prescription is allowed to substitute some other version of the drug if it is cheaper or the only one available.

To understand how antibiotics work you must understand the notion of *resistance*, the ability of some bacteria to escape the effect of the drug. Some of this resistance is natural, because some antibiotics target bacterial properties that some bacteria do not have, such as a key life-support system of the bacterial cell. The worrisome kind of bacterial resistance to antibiotics is the sort passed back and forth among bacteria themselves, such as an enzyme that allows the germ to inactivate the antibiotic molecule. In this way, bacteria can acquire resistance to an antibiotic that had worked well against them in the past.

The largest group of antibiotics is made up of those that attack the cell wall of the microorganism, essentially blowing the germ apart. They work best against rapidly growing bacteria rather than dormant bacteria, because it is the multiplying bacteria that are making new cell walls. These cell-wall drugs are divided into two huge groups: the *penicillins* (and their many offspring) and the *cephalosporins*.

Penicillin was a true miracle drug when it appeared in the 1940s, curing children who would otherwise have died. The original penicillin, termed penicillin G, is still used today, although most bacteria long ago became resistant to it by acquiring an enzyme that inactivates the penicillin molecule before it can destroy the germ. Fortunately for those of us who treat children, the bacteria causing strep throat and the most common variety of impetigo is one of the few still sensitive to penicillin, so we still use this extremely safe drug to treat those infections. Penicillin can be injected into a vein or muscle—the latter typically as a long-acting form that lasts for days—or taken by mouth. The oral form of the drug is called *penicillin V*, often shortened to PenV. It is one of the cheapest of antibiotics, must be stored in the refrigerator, and a child typically takes it two to four times per day for one to two weeks.

The original penicillin had no activity against several bacteria that often cause respiratory and urinary tract infections. Chemists soon tweaked the molecule to produce drugs that did—*ampicillin* and *amoxicillin*. The latter medicine is overall the most commonly used antibiotic for children. When some bacteria became resistant, however, amoxicillin was combined with another agent to produce another widely used and very useful drug with the most common brand name of *Augmentin*.

The first cousins of penicillins are the antibiotics termed cephalosporins. Unlike the penicillins, only a few of which we use today, cephalosporins form an enormous group of antibiotics, one commonly used for children. They are also much more expensive than penicillin. Cephalosporins share with penicillin a general mode of action—they kill bacteria by destroying a sensitive microorganism's protective cell wall. Also like penicillin, many bacteria are no longer sensitive, having found ways to escape the effects of the drug.

Chemists, in their continuing efforts to thwart the germs and widen the spectrum of bacteria sensitive to antibiotics, have altered the original cephalosporin molecule to produce several generations of the drug family. Doctors use representatives of all of these to treat infections in children. Intravenous forms of cephalosporins are commonly used to treat serious infections in hospitalized children. Children brought to the emergency department or doctor's office often receive one of the oral forms. The first-generation version of *cefalexin* (Keflex or Duricef) is very useful for skin infections; its second-generation relative, *cefuroxime* (Ceftin) is often used for respiratory or ear infections. Doctors generally use third-generation varieties, of which there are many expensive versions (Suprax, Vantin), for particularly difficult or unusual infections, such as from a highly resistant germ.

Ceftriaxone (Rocephin) is not an oral antibiotic. However, it is a third-generation cephalosporin that lasts so long in the body a child can get an injection that will last twenty-four hours. Since getting small children to take large doses of oral medicine is often challenging, doctors use ceftriaxone if they wish to guarantee a good level of antibiotic in a child's system. It is widely used both for this reason and because it kills many bacteria that commonly infect children.

There are now even fourth-generation cephalosporins, medications pharmaceutical chemists have constructed in their race to keep one step ahead of the germs, as well as drugs that combine aspects of cephalosporins with penicillins. These drugs are beyond the scope of our discussion, but you may find your child needing one of these if she has an infection from a particularly resistant microbe. Nearly all of these cephalosporins must be injected into the vein, and therefore usually require the child to be in the hospital.

Azithromycin (Zithromax) is currently the most commonly used member of another group of antibiotics, other examples of which are *clarithromycin* (Biaxin) and *erythromycin* (E-mycin, EES). Doctors often use these drugs to treat respiratory and skin infections in children, particularly if they cannot take penicillins or cephalosporins. They also are used to treat whooping cough and the bacterium that causes stomach ulcers. The chief advantage of azithromycin over the others is that it can be given only once a day and for only half the duration most oral antibiotics require. It also causes less stomach upset than was common with its older cousins.

Sulfonamide antibiotics are the oldest class of all, older even than penicillin, and we still sometimes use them in treating children. Sulfa eye drops (Sulamyd) are often used for conjunctivitis (pinkeye). The most common oral variety is actually a mixture of sulfa with a related antibiotic, *tremethoprim*. The combination comes in several brand names, the most common being Septra and Bactrim. It is often used to treat urinary tract infections and sometimes respiratory infections.

Antibiotics are powerful, useful, and sometimes lifesaving medicines. Even though their safety profile is generally excellent compared to other drugs, there are aspects we should be cautious of if we use them. In the treatment of children, most antibiotics kill many other bacteria besides those causing the infection. This is not a good thing, since our bodies rely on normal, "friendly" bacteria living in our intestines to do several important things for us, such as crowd out "unfriendly" bacteria and make an important vitamin we cannot make ourselves, vitamin K. Although a child's body restores its normal microbiological ecology soon after the antibiotics are stopped, prolonged use of these drugs can lead to harmful changes in what we call the *bacterial flora* of a child's body.

There is another reason doctors are careful prescribing antibiotics. As you read above, many disease-causing bacteria are becoming resistant to antibiotic action, and widespread use of them accelerates this process because it selects for the resistant strains by killing off the competition, the antibiotic-sensitive ones. This happens both in a person's own body and in the wider environment; antibiotic-resistant "super-bacteria" pose a risk to all of us.

ANTIVIRAL MEDICATIONS

Antibiotics kill bacteria, not viruses. This is unfortunate, because viral illness is especially common in young children. The time may be coming when we can treat the many viruses that cause colds and flu, but as of this moment we have only two kinds of medicine that have any effect upon viruses, and they do not kill the most common ones. One drug is called *acyclovir* (Zovirax), and it only works against several members of the *herpes virus* family. Acyclovir is useful in treating children with widespread sores in the mouth from herpes virus or who have varicella virus, the closely related virus that causes chickenpox. The second agent, *oseltamivir* (Tamiflu), has some effect on the influenza virus, but only if the medication is given early in the course of the illness; it has little effect on an established disease.

ANTIFEVER MEDICATIONS

Children get fevers frequently, usually from infections. Many parents notice that fever makes their child listless and unwilling to eat or drink much, which can lead to dehydration. Rapid rise in temperature can also provoke seizures in some toddlers. It is important for parents to know, however, that although a very high, sustained fever can cause injury to the brain, this is a very rare occurrence. Fever itself causes no harm; it is, after all, part of the body's natural response to infection. Fever does make many children miserable, though, so treating fever is a cornerstone of supportive care even if it does nothing about the cause of the fever. Antifever medicines can be obtained without a prescription. Since they are so important for childhood diseases, it is useful for parents to know how they work.

The first antifever medicine was aspirin. Its discovery, from willow tree bark, was a milestone in modern medicine. Aspirin was used in treating children for many years, but its association with *Reye's Syndrome*, a rare and frequently fatal pediatric disease, makes it too dangerous to treat fever in children under age twelve.

The two standard antifever medications are *acetaminophen* (Tylenol, many others) and *ibuprofen* (Advil, Motrin, many others), both of which come as tablets or liquid with age-appropriate doses written on the box or bottle. Both drugs are effective in treating fever, but they work in somewhat different ways. The main difference is that, whereas acetaminophen works principally in the brain, resetting the body's "thermostat," ibuprofen also has profound effects on the rest of the body besides working in the brain to control fever. You will read more about this below.

ANTI-INFLAMMATORY MEDICATIONS

Inflammation is a common and important response of the body to many kinds of stress and irritation. Unfortunately, inflammation also causes such unpleasant things as fever, pain, swelling, and itching. Severe inflammation can be life-threatening. Doctors use several kinds of medications to lessen the effects of inflammation, both to relieve the symptoms and to dampen the body's inflammatory response to a host of irritants. Thus anti-inflammatory drugs can be both specific treatments or a component of supportive care.

Ibuprofen is the most commonly used anti-inflammatory medicine. It works by blocking the production of several potent chemicals in certain of the body's cells—chemicals that act on other cells to cause the symptoms of inflammation, particularly swelling and pain. It is effective for reducing the inflammation (and the pain) caused by such things as twisted knees and sprained ankles.

Other kinds of inflammation, such as severe skin rashes from poison ivy or hives, are not helped by ibuprofen. The most effective drug for these inflammations is one of the class called *corticosteroids*, which are analogs of the hormone *cortisol* naturally made by our adrenal glands. Steroid medicines have nearly as many varieties as antibiotics, but a good way to classify them is by distinguishing among those injected into the body, those taken by mouth, and those smeared on the skin as a cream or ointment. Regardless, they all work the same way—by blocking certain *pro-inflammatory cells* in the body from releasing powerful substances that lead to all the symptoms of inflammation. Ibuprofen does this to some extent, but steroids are much more effective at doing it.

The hallmark of an inflammatory rash is itching, often accompanied by clear fluid weeping from the skin that dries as a crust. Poison ivy is a good example of this type of rash. Steroid cream, available over the counter in its weaker forms or by prescription for its stronger versions, goes directly to the inflamed area to put out the inflammatory fire, relieving the itching and drying the rash as it does so. Inflammation that extends widely over the body, or that causes other body areas to swell and ache, such as the joints or the throat, needs more than cream. Oral steroids, the most common forms being *prednisone* or *prednisolone*, are very effective for this. If the inflammation is severe, the doctor uses injected steroids, such as *methylprednisolone* or *dexamethasone*. The latter medicine is very effective for croup, for example.

You will read more about drug reactions and side effects later in the chapter. Doctors use steroids, however, with special caution. Even though these medicines are quite safe in the short-term, they can cause a host of serious problems if used for prolonged periods of time—weeks to months.

ASTHMA AND WHEEZING MEDICATIONS

I have used as examples children with asthma. This is because asthma and wheezing are extremely common complaints in children. These drugs are the second-most frequently prescribed medications for children after antibiotics. From a practical perspective, whether or not the doctor calls your child's breathing difficulties asthma, the medicines we use to treat the symptoms are similar for all kinds of wheezing. Wheezing comes from bands of muscle that surround the small airways in the lungs; when the muscles contract, the bands constrict. This closes down the airways, making it difficult for the air to get out and resulting in the high-pitched wheezing sound of the air whistling past these tiny obstructions.

The most important drugs for treating wheezing are those that make the constricting bands of muscles relax and allow the airway to return to normal size. The class of drugs that does this is called *beta-agonists*, and the most commonly used one in children is *albuterol* (Ventolin, Proventil, many others). The easiest, most effective way to give the drug is to deliver it right to the airways in the form of an aerosolized mist the child breathes. Many parents who have children with a wheezing problem have a machine to do this at home, a *nebulizer*, so they are ready immediately when their child has breathing troubles.

More convenient than a nebulizer is a pocket-sized, *metered-dose inhaler* (an MDI or "puffer") that uses a propellant to shoot the albuterol down into the child's lungs. The nebulizer requires little cooperation from the child; in contrast, the MDI requires the child to inhale at the right moment. We have plastic chambers that plug into the MDI that allow MDI use even in toddlers, but this is more difficult to get right than using a nebulizer.

Albuterol is first-line therapy for wheezing, whether the wheezing is caused by asthma or a respiratory virus infection. Children with asthma, however, have substantial airway inflammation as part of their problem; we treat this with anti-inflammatory drugs, primarily steroids. If a child is seriously ill with asthma, we give the steroids by mouth or in the vein, usually as a "pulse" of five days to avoid the long-term side effects. Steroids can also be given right to the trouble zone in the form of either a nebulized drug (Pulmacort) or as an MDI (Flovent and many others). Inhaled steroids do not cause the bodywide side effects of steroids taken by mouth or in the vein because they do not penetrate past the airways in significant amounts. This is fortunate, because steroids work best if the child takes them every day, regardless of symptoms.

Many children with asthma need daily preventative doses of both beta-agonists and steroids. To make it easier for children to take these medications, many doctors prescribe an inhaler that combines in one puff both a long-acting albuterol-type drug and a steroid. Brand-named Advair, this approach is becoming increasingly popular because of the convenience of having two drugs in one dose.

Asthma experts often use a therapeutic approach of a combination of several medications that work in different ways, always with the goal of reducing the airway constriction and inflammation that is the hallmark of the disorder. Beta-agonists plus inhaled steroids is one example of this, but we have others. An oral drug called *montelukast* (Singulair) dampens the inflammatory response as does an inhaled medicine called *cromolyn* (Intal); another inhaled drug, *ipratropium bromide* (Atrovent) reduces the amount of mucus in the airway. Depending upon how severe a child's symptoms are, doctors may prescribe one or more of these to attack the asthma from several directions.

ALLERGY MEDICATIONS

Allergies are common among children, although perhaps not as common as nonphysicians think they are. It is certainly true that parents often ascribe a wide variety of vague symptoms and complaints in children to "allergies." Physicians were once more prone to do this, too, particularly when the biological basis for allergies was being worked out four or five decades ago. These days doctors are more precise with the term. This is important, because the drug treatment for allergies can be complicated and often must last for years.

To understand how allergy therapies work, you need to understand a little about how allergic reactions occur in the body, because all treatments are designed to block or at least reduce those cellular reactions. Immunologists—the experts—have divided allergic reactions into several categories. For a parent with a wheezing, sneezing child, the most important of these is the immediate response to a substance, an *allergen*, the child is exposed to.

Those people who are allergic to something have special cells, *mast cells*, primed to go off when the cell encounters a particular allergen. Not surprisingly, mast cells are usually found in the nasal passages, the skin, and the lungs. The cells are stuffed full of substances, the most important of which is *histamine*, that the cell releases to the surrounding tissues when triggered by the allergen. Histamine has several well-known effects, all of which correlate with typical allergic symptoms. It makes the tiny blood vessels leak fluid, leading to such problems as hives in the skin, a runny nose, and sneezing. Down in the lungs, histamine causes constriction of the airways, leading to cough and wheezing and increased fluid and mucus in the airways. The extent of these symptoms is variable with the individual child, more or less correlating with how many primed mast cells the child has and where they are located.

The oldest medications for allergy treatment are antihistamines. There are many, many of these, in both prescription and over-the-counter versions, but the standard, prototypic one is *diphenhydramine* (Benadryl). Although it lasts only several hours, it is very effective in blocking the histamine response for most allergic children. However, it has the significant side effect of causing moderate to severe drowsiness. It does this so consistently that doctors often use the drug not as an allergy medicine but as a sleeping aid.

Pharmaceutical chemists solved this problem by devising antihistamines that would not penetrate from the bloodstream to the brain; they still blocked histamine, they just did not cause sleepiness. There are several of these nonsedating antihistamines available, common brand names include Claritin and Zyrtec.

Many, even most of the over-the-counter antihistamines are compounded with other drugs designed to block the effects of histamine on the tissues. The traditional type of this antihistamine is *pseudoephedrine* (Sudafed and many others), which dries up a child's nasal passages by preventing the fluid release histamine causes. Pseudoephedrine, however, has significant side effects, especially for children; it is a potent stimulant, being a precursor to *methamphetamine*, a highly addictive and illegal stimulant. In fact, illicit diversion of pseudoephedrine to the manufacture of methamphetamines has nearly taken it from the over-the-counter market. It has been largely replaced by *phenylephrine* (Sudafed PE and many others), which cannot be made into methamphetamine.

Children with allergies are common. Much more common, however, are children with colds. Accordingly, drug companies have marketed these over-the-counter mixtures of sedating antihistamines and nasal drying agents largely as therapies for cold symptoms. However, pediatric authorities, such as the American Academy of Pediatrics, recommend they not be used for colds because they seldom help much—cold viruses do not affect the system like allergies do—and their side effects can cause problems.

Since allergies, like asthma, cause inflammation of the respiratory tract, we use several of the asthma drugs to treat allergic symptoms. Both steroids (Nasilide, many others) and cromolyn (Nasal-Crom, many others) can be sprayed into the nose and are often effective in controlling an allergic child's runny nose. Of course, it is not always easy to spray things into an uncooperative child's nose, and both of these medicines do not work immediately; they require at least several days before they cause any improvement.

Ever since doctors knew the cellular basis of allergic symptoms, we have tried ways to prevent them in the first place, particularly for those children whose symptoms are truly life-threatening, such as children exquisitely sensitive to bee stings. If we can use skin testing to identify the specific allergens responsible for a child's symptoms, then repeated small injected doses of that allergen can *desensitize* the child's mast cells to it. This does not always work, and weeks and weeks of injections are required, but for some children, desensitization therapy helps dramatically.

STOMACH ACID MEDICATIONS

The stomach is an interesting organ. It houses the second phase of food digestion, after the enzymes in saliva begin the process, and is filled with acid released by cells in its lining. This acid can destroy tissues, including the stomach itself. What prevents destruction of the stomach is its acid-resistant lining. Sometimes, however, the balance between the ability of the stomach lining to contain the acid and the corrosive nature of the stomach contents is disrupted, leading to pain.

More common is backflow of acid from the stomach into the lower part of the *esophagus*, the swallowing tube, a process known as *gastro-esophageal reflux* to doctors—heartburn to everyone else. The reason reflux hurts is that the esophagus does not have the same protective lining the stomach has. If the process of backflow continues, besides chronic pain it can cause long-lasting injury to the esophagus. In children, especially infants, a small or moderate amount of reflux is common, even normal; any parent burping a baby knows that an infant's stomach contents often end up on the parent's shoulder. More severe reflux causes the child pain and sometimes breathing problems and therefore needs treatment.

We can diagnose severe reflux in several ways. We can use an X-ray that looks for swallowed barium going backward up the esophagus; we can used a special probe that measures how much and how often acid is present in the esophagus; or a specialist can actually look at the lower esophagus through an endoscope to see if there are any acid burns present. Severe reflux usually needs surgery to fix.

Much more commonly, doctors use drugs to block stomach acid, allowing the reflux to continue but relieving the pain and acid damage. Since reflux nearly always gets better as a child grows, this is our usual approach. This makes reflux treatment a form of supportive care—we are doing nothing for the reflux itself, merely relieving the symptoms until the problem goes away on its own.

We have two kinds of drugs to block stomach acid production. The older of these, *ranitidine* (Zantac) has been used safely in children for many years and is now even available over the counter. Ranitidine works well most of the time, but we now have a new generation of much more powerful drugs, *omeprazole* (Prilosec and others) and *lansoprazole* (Prevacid and others). These drugs block over 99 percent of stomach acid production. We do not as yet have as much experience treating children with the newer drugs as we have with ranitidine. They appear to be quite safe, although the effect of blocking acid production over the long term—years and years—is unknown.

PAIN MEDICATIONS

Medicines for pain are a pure example of supportive care; they are designed for the comfort of the child and do not by themselves cure anything. Although it was once thought, erroneously, that children do not experience pain in the same way adults do, current pediatric practice is to provide children the same kind of pain relief as adults. Most of the time that can be accomplished using one or both of two of the combination anti-inflammatory and pain-relief medicines described above—acetaminophen and ibuprofen. These usually are all that is needed for simple bumps, bruises, and sprains.

More severe pain, such as from a broken bone, needs stronger medicine, usually from the *narcotic* class of medications. There are many of these, some of which are available in liquid form for children. Of these medications, *codeine* is probably the most frequently prescribed, typically in combination with acetaminophen. It also was once thought dangerous to use these medications in children; research has now shown this not to be true, as long as the medication is dosed correctly.

ATTENTION DEFICIT HYPERACTIVITY DISORDER (ADHD) MEDICATIONS

The number of children diagnosed with ADHD has increased in recent years. It is an area of considerable controversy among physicians, psychologists, educators, and concerned parents. At times it does seem as if any child who is more restless than is deemed normal ends up with this diagnosis. It is not my purpose here to enter this controversy in any way other than to point out that ADHD medicines are now very commonly prescribed in children. Parents whose child's doctor is considering prescribing these drugs should learn about them—how they are believed to work and their side effects—if they are to understand what the doctor is talking about.

Neurotransmitters are substances the brain cells use to communicate with one another, and ADHD appears to be a disorder in this complex communication system. Although the causes for this derangement are, in a general sense, inherited, the inheritance pattern is complicated. The symptoms are also affected by a child's environment, so genetics is not the whole answer. Some of the symptoms of ADHD are restlessness, inattentiveness, and impulsivity. These things make it difficult for an affected child to learn at school, so teachers are often the ones recommending to parents their child be evaluated for ADHD. The diagnosis itself is difficult, and sometimes controversial, because the symptoms overlap normal childhood behavior. In spite of this, doctors do have accepted, standard scales for identifying the extent to which a child's symptoms are normal or not.

The standard drug treatment for ADHD is completely counter-intuitive; children with increased restlessness are treated with stimulants and they become less restless. Many research studies have confirmed that this happens, and also that when the stimulant wears off, the child's hyperactive symptoms return. No one knows how brain stimulants work for children with ADHD. Most researchers presume that they somehow restore the brain's chemical balance by replacing neurotransmitters deficient in the areas of the child's brain that control mood and attentiveness.

The original ADHD drug was *methyphenidate* (Ritalin, Concerta, and others). It is still the most frequently used, although various long-acting preparations have been devised to make its effects last longer between doses. Another commonly used drug is plain amphetamine (Adderall and others). The potential side effects of these drugs are significant, all related to overstimulation of the central nervous and cardiovascular systems. If you and your child's doctor decide to use them, ADHD medications can represent the kind of medicine therapeutic trial you read about previously; children with true ADHD will respond to the stimulant by calming down. Besides your own and your doctor's observations, you should also include your child's teacher's assessment in any decision about how well these medications are working.

ɤ   ɤ   ɤ

All medications, even simple fever drugs, carry some risk. That risk may be small, but it is never zero. When doctors prescribe a medication, they always are considering the risk–benefit question: does the potential benefit to the child outweigh the risk? The most basic risk is that of an unusual allergic reaction to the drug. It is rare, but serious or even life-threatening reactions do happen. This is why one of the key questions we always ask parents in taking a medical history is if their child has ever experienced any drug reactions in the past.

Some drugs are known to be more prone to causing specific side effects. Amoxicillin and ampicillin, for example, commonly cause a nonitching, fine, red rash most prominently seen on a child's chest and abdomen. The rash usually appears several days into therapy. Its cause is unknown, but it does not appear to represent a true allergic reaction to all penicillins—just to ampicillin and amoxicillin. Erythromycin, and especially clarithromycin, is notorious for causing stomach upset. All antibiotics frequently cause diarrhea, probably because of their effect on the normal balance of bacteria that usually grow in the intestines. Often the diarrhea is severe enough that the child must stop taking the antibiotic.

All the other medications you read about carry their own particular risks of side effects. Ibuprofen can cause stomach pains and increase the risk of bleeding. Long-term use of steroids can cause many problems, some of them serious, which is why we use them in as low a dose and for as brief a time as possible. Narcotics can cause excessive sedation and abdominal distress, particularly constipation, nausea, and vomiting. The ADHD drugs are emphatically a class of medicines to be used judiciously because they have powerful effects on the brain.

It is sometimes said that Americans are especially likely to seek a pharmacological solution to all our ills. Your child's doctor should carefully consider whether treatment with a medicine—specific, supportive, or empiric—is the best therapy for your child. It is always appropriate for parents to consider this issue, too, and I hope this chapter will give you the information you need to have that conversation with your child's doctor.

Not all treatments require medicine, and some of the simple medicines are still the most effective. There are many examples of this principal in pediatric practice. The most basic of these, surprisingly not always thought of, is also one that brings to mind a stand-up comedy routine: when an activity causes your child discomfort, stop doing it. Avoidance is usually the safest choice, especially if the contemplated therapy carries risk. Here is a real-life example of what I mean.

I practiced medicine for many years at high altitude. Those of us who live at six or seven thousand feet become acclimated to the relative lack of oxygen, but it is occasionally a problem for visiting tourists. Some years ago I cared for a child who lived near sea level and who developed what is loosely called mountain sickness when his vacationing family drove to over ten thousand feet in altitude. This child's symptoms were difficulty breathing and a buildup of fluid in his lungs, both of which resolved completely when he got the standard therapy of oxygen and specific medication, plus the essential measure of simply coming down to a lower altitude.

All of that was routine; what was not routine was what the child's parents wanted for him. As it happened, this was not the child's first episode of acute mountain sickness—a similar thing had happened to him twice before, just not as severely. On those occasions the child just complained a little to his parents but looked fine, and his symptoms stopped when the family came down the mountain. This time he was worse and needed treatment, which fortunately was effective.

Most parents would have interpreted this third, more ominous event as a sign not to take their child to high altitude; instead, this family wanted prescriptions for portable oxygen and medications to treat excess lung fluid. Adults, particularly mountain sports enthusiasts, make this decision for themselves, but it seemed unfair to me to risk this young child's health (the medicines and oxygen do not always work), when simply staying at a lower altitude fixed the problem. That was my advice to the parents; if doing something nonessential causes trouble every time you do it, stop doing it.

We have many treatments for common pediatric conditions that do not require medicines, and nearly all are extremely low-risk. One is simple lifestyle change, as for the boy with altitude sensitivity. Another example is modifying the environment to improve the symptoms, such as removing curtains and dusty carpets in an allergic child's room. Doctors prescribe allergy medicines, but we will also tell you to do these kinds of safe, low-tech things, too. It is good advice, but it surprises me how many parents would rather substitute a medication for common sense.

There are several common pediatric conditions that are helped by manipulation of a child's diet. A few children have intolerance to foods or even actual allergies to them; sensitivity to the proteins or sugars in cow's milk is a common example. In these children, of course, the answer is to avoid the offending food. Gastroenteritis, often accompanied by diarrhea, is a common pediatric ailment, and small children recovering from this often are helped by restricting their diet for a few days to easily digestible foods; doctors often recommend what is called the "BRAT" diet of bananas, rice, applesauce, and toast, along with plenty of fluids that do not contain large amounts of sugar. A less common but potentially serious condition, *celiac sprue*, is caused by sensitivity to gluten, a substance present in wheat flour. The treatment is to remove gluten from a child's diet.

I hope this chapter has given you useful information about how doctors think of pediatric therapies. Foremost in our minds is always the issue of balancing the chances of the therapy helping the situation against the risk of the treatment; is it truly a matter of "can't hurt, might help," or does the therapy have some potential problems? After all, even the benign BRAT diet can be injurious to a child if parents carry it to extremes and continue it for days and days. The next chapter is about *why* doctors think the way we do and how we were taught to do so.

COMMUNICATION CHECKLIST FOR PARENTS

1. What therapies are the doctor suggesting, and what is the rationale for each?
2. If the doctor recommends no therapy for the underlying problem, but your child has symptoms, is there any supportive care that might help?
3. Are there any risks to the therapies?
4. If the doctor prescribes medications, are there any particular side effects to watch for?
5. If the doctor suggests no therapy, is there a risk in doing nothing?

Chapter 7

WHY WE ARE THIS WAY

How Doctors Are Trained

The previous chapters introduced you to the physician's mental world, showed you how your sick child looks when viewed through a doctor's eyes. This chapter will admit you further into the medical mindset by showing you how doctors got the way we are, how we acquired this particular way of looking at a child's medical problems in the first place. It will give you the kind of deep background information that will acquaint you with your doctor's past mental journey. And the better you understand where she is coming from, the better your conversation with her will go.

The way physicians are trained has not varied much in a century, but the decades before that saw dramatic changes. Most physicians in the nineteenth century received their medical educations in what were called proprietary medical schools. These were schools started as a business enterprise, often, but not necessarily, by doctors. Anyone could start one, since there were no standards of any sort. The success of the school was not a matter of how good the school was, since that quality was then impossible to define anyway, but of how good those who ran it were at attracting paying students.

There were dozens of proprietary medical schools across America. Chicago alone, for example, had fourteen of them at the beginning of the twentieth century. Since these schools were the private property of their owners, who were usually physicians, the teaching curriculum varied enormously between schools. Virtually all the teachers were practicing physicians who taught parttime. Although being taught by actual practitioners is a good thing, at least for clinical subjects, the academic pedigrees and skills of these teachers varied as widely as the schools—some were excellent, some were terrible, and the majority were somewhere in between.

Whatever the merits of the teachers, students of these schools usually saw and treated their first patient after they had graduated because the teaching at these schools consisted nearly exclusively of lectures. Although they might see a demonstration now and then of something practical, in general students sat all day in a room listening to someone tell them about disease rather than showing it to them in actual sick people. There were no laboratories. Indeed, there was no need for them because medicine was taught exclusively as a theoretical construct, and some of its theories dated back to Roman times. It lacked much scientific basis because the necessary science was itself largely unknown at the time.

As the nineteenth century progressed, many of the proprietary schools became affiliated with universities; often several would join to form the medical school of a new state university. The medical school of the University of Minnesota, for example, was established in 1888 when three proprietary schools in Minneapolis merged, with a fourth joining the union some years later. These associations gave medical students some access to aspects of new scientific knowledge, but overall the American medical schools at the beginning of the twentieth century were a hodgepodge of wildly varying quality.

Medical schools were not regulated in any way because medicine itself was largely unregulated. It was not even agreed upon what the practice of medicine actually was; there prevailed at the time among physicians several occasionally overlapping but generally distinct views of what the real causes of disease were. The very definitions of these groups were fiercely contentious, but we have come to label them allopathy, homeopathy, and osteopathy. There was also a substantial group of doctors best labeled empirics—they were willing to use whatever approach seemed to work, irrespective of theory.

The first of these terms, allopathy, was coined to distinguish what was then conventional, mainstream medicine from homeopathy. In brief, whereas allopathic physicians used treatments (often large doses of drugs) designed to produce the opposite effect of a patient's symptoms, homeopathic physicians used a system of giving patients tiny doses of drugs that, in large doses, produced the same symptoms, believing, in their words, that in small doses, "like cures like." Osteopathy, as initially formulated, was based upon the premise that many ailments come from misalignments of the bones, especially the spine. All three of these schools of medical theory suffered from the same defect in that they regarded a symptom, such as fever, as a disease in itself. Thus they believed relieving the symptom was equivalent to curing the disease.

The fundamental problem was that all these warring medical factions had no idea what really caused most diseases; for example, bacteria were only just being discovered and their role in disease was still largely unknown, although this was rapidly changing. Human physiology—how the body works—was only beginning to be investigated. To America's sick patients, none of this made much difference, because virtually none of the medical therapies available at the time did any good, and many of the allopathic treatments, such as large doses of mercury, were even highly toxic to the patient.

One thing an experienced doctor could offer, though, no matter his particular school of medical theory, was a prediction of what would happen to the patient. This is the art of *prognosis*. This is not a trivial thing to offer the sick; it is information about what to expect. In fact, in an era when few treatments did any good and some did serious harm, many patients were grateful just for that assessment of their likely outcome, even though the doctor could do nothing to forestall it. Today's student doctors learn disease prognosis—what will occur with or without treatment—from books and teachers. A century ago that knowledge came from long experience and open-minded observation, whether the doctor was an allopath, a homeopath, or an osteopath.

There were then bitter arguments and rivalries among physicians for other reasons besides their warring theories of disease causation. In that era before experimental science, no one viewpoint could definitely prove another wrong. The chief reason for the rancor, however, was that there were more physicians than there was demand for their services. At a time when few people even went to the doctor, the number of physicians practicing primary care (which is what they all did back then) relative to the population was three times more than it is today. Competition was tough, so tough that the majority of physicians did not even support themselves through the practice of medicine alone; they had some other occupation as well.

In sum, medicine a century ago consisted of an excess of physicians, many of them badly trained, who jealously squabbled with each other as each tried to gain an advantage. Two things changed that medical world into the one we know today: the explosion of scientific knowledge, which finally gave us some insight into how diseases actually behaved in the body, and a revolution in medical education, a revolution wrought by what is known as the Flexner Report.

In 1910 the Carnegie Foundation commissioned Abraham Flexner to visit all 155 medical schools in America (for comparison, there are only 125 today). What he found appalled him; only a few passed muster, principally the Johns Hopkins Medical School, which had been established on the model then prevailing in Germany. That model stressed rigorous training in the new biological sciences with hands-on laboratory experience for all medical students, followed by supervised bedside experience caring for actual sick people.

Flexner's report changed the face of medical education profoundly; eighty-nine of the medical schools he visited closed over the next twenty years, and those remaining structured their curricula into what we have today—a combination of preclinical training in the relevant sciences followed by practical, patient-oriented instruction in clinical medicine. This standard has stood the test of time, meaning the way I was taught in 1974 was essentially unchanged from how my father was taught in 1942.

Meanwhile, the advance of medical science had largely solved the problem of the feuding between kinds of doctors; allopathic, homeopathic, and osteopathic schools adopted essentially the same curriculum. The last of these continues to maintain its own schools, of which there are twenty-three in the United States, and to grant its own degree—the Doctor of Osteopathy (DO), rather than the Doctor of Medicine (MD). In virtually all respects, however, and most importantly in the view of state licensing boards, the skills, rights, and privileges of holders of the two degrees are equivalent.

So how does one train to be a physician? The first step is to obtain a four-year undergraduate degree at a college or university. This was the most fundamental change in post-Flexner medical training; before that time, many medical schools had little or no requirement for previous education, some not even demanding a high school diploma. Today the prospective physician's baccalaureate degree can be in anything (mine happens to be in history and religion), but all medical schools require premedical course work in biology, chemistry, biochemistry, physics, and often mathematics. As a result of these science-heavy requirements, most premedical students choose to major in one of the sciences.

The next step is to gain admission to medical (or osteopathic) school. This traditionally has been a difficult thing to accomplish, although admission statistics for individual schools are hard to interpret because virtually all students apply to several schools, often more than ten. In general, a medical school applicant's overall chances of being admitted to medical school has fluctuated between 25 and 35 percent over the last several decades. One thing that has changed is drop-out rate. Fifty years ago, many students did not complete the course; these days, drop-out rates are extremely low.

Medical school generally lasts four years, at the end of which time the graduate is properly addressed as "doctor." However, the new doctor is one in name only, because no state will allow her to practice medicine independently without further training. Medical licenses are in fact granted by the individual states, and their requirements vary, but all demand at least one year of supervised on-the-job training beyond medical school. Fifty years ago, many physicians stopped their training after doing that single year of training—called an internship—because that was all a physician needed to obtain a medical license and begin working as a general practitioner. These days virtually no one stops after one year, because nearly all physicians require more training just to find a job. You will still hear doctors in their first year out of medical school referred to as interns, but the term does not mean much now.

Medical students receive a standard training curriculum that varies little between the various medical schools; this is enforced by the organization that accredits these schools. Toward the end of their four years, however, students generally do get some freedom to select courses geared toward what specialty they choose for their residency, the term for the several years of practical training they get after medical school. The usage comes from the fact that medical residents once actually lived in the hospital; these days, even though resident workweeks average eighty hours or so, no one literally lives in the hospital.

Residencies come in the standard broad categories of areas of expertise like internal medicine, pediatrics, surgery, and obstetrics and gynecology, as well as specialties like radiology, neurology, dermatology, and psychiatry. There are in total twenty-four recognized medical specialties, each of which sets its own requirements for the residents training in their respective fields. Medical science has expanded sufficiently that a medical student who wishes to specialize in not being a specialist—that is, who wants to do general work—must do a residency in family practice.

Residency lasts from three to five years after medical school, depending upon the specialty. At the end of training, the resident takes an examination. Passing it makes her "board-certified" in the field; someone who has completed the residency requirement but has not yet passed (or has failed) the examination is called "board-eligible." Some physicians choose to continue their training even further beyond residency, to subspecialize in things like cardiology or hematology; you will read about these specialties in a later chapter.

The person you encounter when you bring your child to her doctor's appointment has thus spent at least eleven years getting ready to meet you: four years in college, four years in medical school, and three to five years in residency. That person has also spent much of that time being initiated, perhaps indoctrinated, into a culture, a worldview, that is shared by most physicians. It is a culture foreign to that of many nonphysicians. Its attributes come primarily from the way physicians have been trained since Flexner's reforms of medical education a century ago. Knowing about this time-honored system will help you understand your child's physician, and understanding improves communication.

In spite of all its scientific underpinnings, medicine is not really a science; rather, it is an art guided by science. Medical students spend long hours learning about the science of the body, but they really do not become doctors until they have learned the art at the bedside from experienced clinicians. Medical practice is called practice for a reason; we learn it by practicing it in a centuries-old apprenticeship system, which is really what a residency is. As we do so, and again, in spite of the scientific trappings, we imbibe ways of thinking, of talking, and of doing that are as old as Hippocrates. The rest of this chapter will show you that aspect of medicine. Seeing it is fundamental for your understanding of what doctors do and why.

Although physicians learn at the feet of their elders—the experienced practitioners—a young doctor's peers also heavily influence his training, and through that, his outlook; resident culture is important. Residency is an intense experience that comes at a time in life when most new doctors are relatively young and still evolving their adult characters. In a manner similar to military training, residency throws young people together for lengthy, often emotion-laden duty stints in the hospital. Not surprisingly, and also like military servicepeople, residents often form personal bonds from this shared experience that last for the rest of their lives. Most physicians carry vivid memories from their residency for the duration of their careers.

Recent regulations have limited the maximum number of hours a resident may work each week. These rules came from two sources. One was the common-sense observation that tired residents cannot learn or work well. Common sense, however, cannot change hidebound traditions; what really changed resident work hours was a famous court case in New York (the Libby Zion case), involving a girl who died under the care of overworked residents.

The particulars of that case did not clearly establish that resident fatigue caused Libby's death, but the uproar started a sea of change in how residents are trained.

The mandated maximum of an eighty-hour workweek is still long by any standard, but it had been much longer, and many of today's doctors (myself included) trained under the old system when 110 hours or more per week was not uncommon, with perhaps the gift of every third Sunday off. My own residency program director told us, intending no irony: "The main problem with being on-call only every other night is that you miss half the interesting patients." So, like garrulous ex-Marines, doctors swap tales of the time that, although brief in comparison to a lifelong career, was extraordinarily important in forming their professional behavior. Generalizations are tricky, especially when applied to such a diverse group of people as resident physicians. This caveat aside, parents who understand something about resident culture will gain useful insights into why many physicians think and act the way that we do.

Residents have come through a pathway that generally fosters intense competition and that values academic achievement above all else. In recent years, medical schools and residency programs have, to varying degrees, tried to emphasize the importance of more humanistic skills like empathy and compassion, and the specialty of pediatrics has been among the leaders in doing this. However, it remains true that physicians are the products of a system that rewards those who excel at competing with their colleagues at how much information one can learn, remember, and then produce when asked for it by a superior.

Resident culture encourages young doctors to appear and act all-knowing and self-confident even when they are not. This skill is often called "roundsmanship" and is inculcated from early on in their training. Residents get much of their teaching during the time-honored ritual of rounds, in which a team of residents and their supervising physician walk around to their patients' rooms, pausing at each doorway to discuss the case. The discussion typically begins with the resident presenting the patient's problem and the resident's plan to deal with it to the assembled group, following which the supervising physician often grills the resident about the case. Residents adept at roundsmanship are quick thinkers and have rapid recall of pertinent facts. Master roundsmen, however, are best characterized as fearless when clueless—they appear assured and in control of the situation even when they are not.

I am exaggerating a little for effect, of course, but my point is to show you how years and years of this kind of environment affect most doctors to some extent. Such a background can cause doctors to seem defensive when questioned, for example by a parent, because doctors spend their formative years defending what they are doing to both their peers and to their exacting teachers. It can also make it difficult for a doctor to admit he does not know what to do with a patient, since physicians are conditioned to regard that admission as a real defeat. This attitude is encapsulated in the saying, often applied to surgeons but relevant to all physicians: "Seldom wrong, never in doubt."

Sayings like this are common in medicine, and the rest of the chapter will use these venerable chestnuts of wisdom to illustrate why doctors are the way we are. We are steeped in aphorisms from our first days of medical school, often beginning with some version of what the dean told my father on his first day: "Look at the man (because in those days nearly all medical students were men) on either side of you—neither of them will finish." These days nearly all medical students graduate, but the culture of intense competition persists. This is partly from habit, but also because the top medical students get the top residency positions, and medical students always want to be at the top of whatever list they are on.

There are many illustrative medical sayings, but I will focus on three categories: diagnostic advice, therapeutic advice, and advice about how to live, how to be a good physician. This way of understanding and teaching medicine truly is thousands of years old; one of the oldest medical texts is the *Aphorisms* of Hippocrates, a fascinating compilation that nonphysicians also find interesting and instructive.

Chapter 5 described for you the process of forming a differential diagnosis, of making a list of possibilities ranked in order of probability. Some of the first aphorisms a fledgling doctor learns are those relating to diagnosis. Several of these share a common theme, which is to keep it simple. Medical students and residents are naturally inclined to consider complicated and esoteric diagnoses rather than simple ones because, in the game of roundsmanship, the clever and exotic answer is a good way to show off to your teachers and your fellow residents how much you know. Few points accrue to those with mundane and therefore boring solutions listed in their differential diagnosis. Here are some bits of cautionary wisdom about that tendency.

Common things are common.
When you hear hoofbeats, don't think of zebras.
Something strange is more likely to be a rare manifestation of a
    common thing than a rare thing.
Don't give the patient more than one disease.

These sayings are all variations of the obvious tautology contained in the first one; after all, common things are common because they happen a lot. Therefore, simple statistics indicates that, nearly all the time, your child's ailment will be caused by a common medical problem. The second aphorism is a more colorful way of illustrating the principle. It is one every medical student learns to say, as sagely as possible, when a colleague proposes on rounds some obscure disease as the cause for a child's symptoms. Something obvious should have an obvious explanation.

These first two sayings teach that, when formulating a differential diagnosis, one can certainly include some rare things, a few zebras, on the list. However, these exotic creatures should be at the bottom of the list, far below the common horses at the top. Sometimes, though, the history, physical examination, and laboratory tests do not fit with anything common; all the possibilities seem to be rare entities. What then? How should the physician choose between the zebras?

The standard answer is some version of the third saying; the true answer is most often not a zebra but a horse in disguise. Common things are still common, only sometimes they show themselves in odd ways. Thus residents should learn all the unusual manifestations of common disorders because they are much more likely to encounter a nonstandard version of a standard problem than a nonstandard problem.

The last aphorism is derived from one you see quoted in many fields outside medicine, especially in the sciences. It is a version of what is often called *Occam's razor*, after the medieval philosopher who wrote "Plurality should not be posited without necessity." It stresses that the simplest solution is always the preferred one. When a young doctor is confronted by a child who has a variety of symptoms and physical signs, she should draw up a differential diagnosis list containing items that individually could explain all the findings. In other words, "Don't give the patient two diseases."

Thus, for example, if your son has abdominal pain, cough, and headache, the doctor will search for a single cause for all the complaints. Occam's razor cautions her against concluding that your son has appendicitis, allergies, and migraine as three separate culprits for three different symptoms. Even if she cannot stuff all your child's symptoms into one diagnostic box, she will still try to relate them in some way because it is an unlucky child indeed who gets three random diagnoses at the same time. In our hypothetical example, a somewhat far-fetched way to do this would be to diagnose a primary pneumonia, the severe coughing from which strained his abdominal muscles, and the stress of which triggered his preexisting migraine tendency.

The problem with these admonitions is that sometimes they are incorrect. In diagnosing what is wrong with patients, doctors should keep it simple because common things are common, but uncommon things do happen. Hoof beats may usually come from horses, but sometimes the doctor may find himself on the medical equivalent of the African savannah. Young doctors are also taught a version of this principle, one encapsulated by a sentiment attributed to, among others, H. L. Mencken, George Bernard Shaw, and Mark Twain: that every complicated problem has a simple, elegant solution, which, in spite of Occam's razor, is wrong. And sometimes patients do indeed have two diseases.

The cases in chapter 1 are excellent examples of the inherent tension between these opposing diagnostic principles. Although I presented the stories to you as instances in which parents and doctors did not communicate, did not hear each other, they also serve as examples of what happens when doctors, especially when busy, rely too much on the statistical truth that common things are the most likely explanation.

In the first case, the child with breathing difficulties, two successive doctors decided the problem was croup, even though there were several atypical features, particularly the very sudden onset, that should have served as red flags, indicators that this case was perhaps really an uncommon thing rather than an uncommon manifestation of a common thing. The doctors finally did figure it out after the story got stranger and stranger—and the symptoms looked less and less like ordinary croup—but it took several visits to the doctor to reach that point.

On the surface, the second case in the chapter appears to violate the diagnostic maxim of not giving the patient two diseases. The basketball-playing adolescent had two disorders, not one, and one of them was a very uncommon disease. This is not as bad an infraction of the rules as it first seems, though, since these two problems were related in a chain of causation; the abnormal heart rhythm caused the boy to faint, strike his head, and suffer a concussion.

The third story in the chapter, the boy who fell from his bike and landed on a rattlesnake, is similar to the second case in that all the symptoms can be related to each other. However, I cannot recall a case that better illustrates the counterprinciple to hoof beats and zebras—sometimes very strange things happen, and we doctors need to keep our minds open to the weirdest of possibilities.

This set of medical sayings teaches us what a delicate mental balancing act medical diagnosis is. Even though doctors should prefer the simplest solution to a complex problem and search for a usual explanation for an unusual set of symptoms, we should also keep our minds open to the possible exceptions. As a parent, you can be enormously helpful to your child's doctor in this process; understanding how the medical diagnostic mind tends to work, you can do your part to prevent the doctor from chasing either a false zebra or a masquerading horse down the wrong diagnostic path.

Medical students and residents also hear many aphorisms about therapies, about how to treat patients. Some of these sayings apply to therapies once the doctor knows the diagnosis; others apply more to advice about the therapeutic trial, about trying something to see if it helps even if the diagnosis is obscure. The sayings come in two opposing viewpoints, yet each is an example of the philosophical tension inherent in the practice of medicine. These viewpoints can be described as confident advice to forge ahead versus cautionary advice to hold back and wait. As you will read, the second tradition is the older and richer of the two. First, here are two well-known sayings counseling an aggressive approach:

A chance to cut is a chance to cure.
When in doubt, cut it out.

It is the surgeons who have the reputation in medicine for being the most likely to push for action; after all, surgeons operate—it is what they do. But this viewpoint is not confined to surgeons; many physicians are inclined to regard treatment as superior to no treatment in most situations. American physicians seem especially more prone than European physicians to bias in favor of treatment, perhaps reflecting our traditional penchant for action, for intervention. This is a tradition dating back to colonial times, when the famous physician (and signer of the Declaration of Independence) Benjamin Rush advocated heroic, misguided, and even lethal therapies. Studies have suggested that this tendency, one still with us, is not forced upon American patients; the aggregate can-do attitude of American physicians largely reflects what Americans want from their doctors. In general, doctors get recognition for doing things, not for the opposite.

Doctors' rationales for their prescribed therapies are not always very scientific. Often they are based on anecdotes or tradition. In the former situation, a doctor believes a treatment is a good one because he knows of, or has read about, patients who have gotten the treatment and improved; in the latter, the treatment is simply what we have always done, sometimes for quite shaky reasons. One of the great scientific breakthroughs of the past fifty years is the widespread use of what are called controlled, randomized clinical trials, in which a treatment is tested uniformly in a group of patients, usually against the results of either no treatment or some other treatment, and with neither the patient nor the treating doctor knowing what the patient is getting until the study is over.

Another common medical saying confronts this issue directly:

The pathway to Hell is not paved with good intentions; it is paved with uncontrolled clinical trials.

The sentiment means that doctors' biases, often derived from anecdotal reports of what seemed to help in the past, affect the therapies we give our patients. It is a natural introduction to the far larger body of medical aphorisms advising caution and restraint in treating patients. Here are some examples of the many I have heard over the years, the first of which comes from Hippocrates, the father of Western medicine.

> Life is short, the art [of medicine] is long, opportunity fleeting, experience delusive, judgment difficult.
> First, do no harm.
> Tincture of time is the best medicine.
> Do not attempt to make a patient better faster than it took the patient to become ill.
> The worst enemy of good is better.
> If it takes more than ten minutes of discussion to decide if a patient needs an operation, it is best not to operate.
> A surgeon knows how to operate, a good surgeon knows when to operate, and an excellent surgeon knows when not to operate.

In spite of our temptation to do something, anything, to help make patients better, by far the stronger tradition in medicine is to do nothing. The reason for this is simple: for most of its history, medicine had next to nothing useful with which to treat anything. Worse, those treatments in vogue, things like bleeding and purging, were often quite toxic and were the exact opposite of what the patient really needed. People noticed that patients often did worse with these treatments than with no treatment at all. Oliver Wendell Holmes Sr., a physician as well as a popular author of the mid-nineteenth century, wrote of that era's treatments: "I firmly believe that if the whole *materia medica* [meaning its medicines] could be sunk to the bottom of the sea, it would be all the better for mankind and all the worse for the fishes."

Observations such as this provided much of the original appeal of homeopathy, although Holmes himself wrote a denunciation of the theory. However, even though homeopathy might or might not help, it certainly did not kill the patient. Samuel Hahnemann, the founder of homeopathy two hundred years ago, had the opportunity to treat many patients during a cholera epidemic in Germany. Whereas his therapies were innocuous, those of his mainstream medical competitors were not; they purged their patient with powerful laxatives and bled pints and pints of blood from them. Since cholera kills through dehydration from massive diarrhea, it is no surprise that Hahnemann's patients did no worse than those who got no treatment at all. In contrast, those treated by the other doctors died in huge numbers.

The sayings above show you that, in spite of the toxic therapies of the last century and before, physicians, even American physicians, have always advised caution. Hippocrates' advice counsels against the folly of doctors believing they know exactly what is going on inside a patient. Interestingly, he also admonishes us to beware of the clinical anecdote; just because we once did something and the patient improved does not mean that the improvement was a result of our therapy, because "experience [is] delusive."

The aphorism "first, do no harm"—*primum non nocere* in Latin—is a widely quoted bit of ancient advice many nonphysicians have heard or read, perhaps because its wisdom applies to much of life outside medicine. Indeed, one might call it the prime directive of both medicine and of life. Although our treatments do sometimes cause the patient harm—side effects and complications happen—on balance we should ensure that the chances of benefit outweigh the risks of harm.

The third saying uses the common medical expression "tincture of time," by which we mean "watchful waiting." The notion is fundamental to how we look upon what medical practice actually consists of: we should not confuse such expectant observation with doing nothing. It sounds a little paradoxical, but treating with the ancient remedy of tincture of time is still a form of treatment. Sometimes we wait because the time is not yet right for treatment, yet we must be vigilant because, as Hippocrates wrote, the "opportunity [is] fleeting."

The next expression on the list counsels patience when we do decide to use a treatment. There are exceptions, of course, but it is a good general principle that anything that took a long time to come will probably take a long time to go, so we should patiently wait for our carefully considered treatments to have a result before we are tempted to try something else.

Next comes the medical equivalent of the old lament that one should have quit while ahead, one should not fix something that is not broken—doctors should leave well enough alone when things are going reasonably well. I have seen many instances where good's worst enemy truly was better. A simple example is readjusting a functioning intravenous line to make it run even better and as a result dislodging the device so that the child needs to have a new needle stick to replace it. A more drastic example is a child who has a second heart operation to improve upon some esoteric and, in retrospect, unimportant aspect of the first one's result, only to suffer a complication from the second procedure.

The last two sayings on the list are rejoinders that thoughtful surgeons say to their more aggressive colleagues. The fact that they also say them to surgical residents shows that not all surgeons enthusiastically espouse the earlier aphorism that "a chance to cut is a chance to cure." After all, although many medical treatments have risks, it is the surgical ones that typically carry the highest chance of what physicians euphemistically call "therapeutic misadventures."

These sayings, and there are many others like them, demonstrate the constant tug-of-war physicians experience between calls for action and recommendations on behalf of inaction. Disconcerting as it can be to parents of sick children, this dialectic is a good thing because it continually forces us to weigh the potential benefits of what we do against the risk of doing it. There are a few sayings that unite these opposing tendencies. Here is one such synthesis, often called "Loeb's rules," after Robert Loeb, a famous physician who taught generations of residents at Columbia University's College of Physicians and Surgeons.

> If what you are doing is doing good, keep doing it.
> If what you are doing is not doing good, stop doing it.
> If you do not know what to do, do nothing.
> Never make the treatment worse than the disease.

Loeb's list has several variations, sometimes including an additional, tongue-in-cheek rule: "Try your best to keep your patient out of the operating room." (Doctor Loeb was not a surgeon.)

Throughout their training, medical students and residents are steeped in these nuggets of wisdom and bon mots from their medical elders, sayings often called "pearls." As teaching tools, they serve as a kind of shorthand for how to reason and solve patient problems as a doctor. Since so many of them date from long ago, they also function as a mini-tour through medical history.

There is, however, an entirely different class of venerable medical sayings that teach about medicine as a way of life, and thus how the resident should live her life as a doctor. It is good for parents to read about these sayings, too, because it will give you considerable insight into the moral culture physicians are taught along with their medical skills. Most of these are inspirational exhortations, often from famous past physicians, and are therefore favorites of medical school graduation speakers. Like all such formulations, they represent ideals doctors should aim at, even if we do not live up to their lofty precepts.

These sayings come from the worldview that medicine is not a job; rather, it is a profession, an ancient and honorable calling. As such, it ought to carry with it obligations along with its privileges. And it does have privileges, something most easily recognized by the fact that practicing medicine is an activity regulated by each of the states in the public interest. In the nineteenth century, nearly anyone could call themselves a physician and treat the sick; now this right is restricted to those licensed by the individual state governments.

The moral obligations of physicians date at least to the founder. Many medical students still swear at their graduation the Oath of Hippocrates. The original text does contain a few odd things—after all, it is nearly twenty-five hundred years old—so many schools use a slightly updated version. A commonly used version today was adapted in 1964 by a medical school dean, Louis Lasagna.

> I swear to fulfill, to the best of my ability and judgment, this covenant:
> I will respect the hard-won scientific gains of those physicians in whose steps I walk, and gladly share such knowledge as is mine with those who are to follow.
> I will apply, for the benefit of the sick, all measures required, avoiding those twin traps of overtreatment and therapeutic nihilism.
> I will remember that there is art to medicine as well as science, and that warmth, sympathy, and understanding may outweigh the surgeon's knife or the chemist's drug.
> I will not be ashamed to say "I know not," nor will I fail to call in my colleagues when the skills of another are needed for a patient's recovery.
> I will respect the privacy of my patients, for their problems are not disclosed to me that the world may know. Most especially must I tread with care in matters of life and death.
> If it is given me to save a life, all thanks. But it may also be within my power to take a life; this awesome responsibility must be

faced with great humbleness and awareness of my own
frailty. Above all, I must not play at God.

I will remember that I do not treat a fever chart, a cancerous
growth, but a sick human being, whose illness may affect the
person's family and economic stability. My responsibility
includes these related problems, if I am to care adequately for
the sick.

I will prevent disease whenever I can, for prevention is preferable
to cure.

I will remember that I remain a member of society, with special
obligations to all my fellow human beings, those sound of
mind and body as well as the infirm.

If I do not violate this oath, may I enjoy life and art, respected
while I live and remembered with affection thereafter. May I
always act so as to preserve the finest traditions of my calling
and may I long experience the joy of healing those who seek
my help.

There are several key aspects to the oath, concepts that Dr.
Lasagna preserved from the original in his updated version. The
oath implies throughout the concept of duty and the occasional
need for sacrifice. There is the notion that medicine is a learned profession, with an obligation to share knowledge with society. Medicine has ancient and honorable traditions, things which must be
respected and upheld. Nonphysicians who see doctors as hidebound
and secretive in the way they do things thus may rightfully find
some of the roots for these things in the oath itself.

The oath also admonishes physicians to treat all patients
equally, irrespective of social or financial status, and to keep all
information about their medical and social conditions confidential.
There is an implied obligation to treat the poor without expecting
payment, since the physician has "special obligations to all . . .
human beings." Most importantly, the oath charges physicians to

treat the patient, not the disease—to see the humanity of the person with the disease.

Finally, the oath implies that physicians should be held to stricter standards of conduct in all matters, not just medical ones. This viewpoint continues today in quite practical ways. For example, virtually all states require physicians, when they renew their medical licenses, to report to the state all legal judgments against them beyond minor traffic offenses. This requirement includes everything, such as drug convictions, that could affect a physician's ability to practice medicine. Thus a charge of reckless driving could lose a doctor her medical license, and a charge of drunk driving, even if the doctor is not on duty, will certainly result in the state requiring her to enroll in a closely monitored alcohol treatment program if she wishes to keep her conditional privileges to practice. I know of one vacationing physician who lost his medical license for assaulting a game warden in an argument over fishing regulations. Physicians are held to a higher standard of conduct. Young residents are taught that this is what society expects.

> Some patients, though conscious that their condition is perilous, recover their health simply through their contentment with the goodness of the physician.
> Being a physician means living more lives than your own.
> To cure sometimes, to relieve often, to comfort always.

The first of these sayings comes from Hippocrates himself. It stresses the importance of the bond between physician and patient, the aspect of trust that the good physician must first earn and then respect and keep. It implies that, whatever the grave circumstances of the clinical situation, the physician must maintain a supportive demeanor, and that simple faith in the physician has healing powers of its own.

The second aphorism continues the theme of medical practice

being something larger than the individual doctor. As a physician, you are vicariously but still deeply involved in the welfare of fellow humans. The words imply that this is a joy, a blessing to the physician, but that it is still something that must be treated reverently in recognition of the privilege it represents.

The third saying is an old one, and is something young doctors frequently see inscribed in book dedications, on graduation programs, and over medical school doorways. It teaches the crucial importance of providing relief of both physical and psychic discomfort in our patients. At the time it was written, of course, "to cure sometimes" might easily have been formulated as "to cure hardly ever."

Most of the sayings you have read thus far are unattributed, handed down in the profession from teacher to student. Most of the following sayings have a known author. Many are from one of the founders of modern medical practice, William Osler. He is so quotable that he is a perennial favorite of graduation speakers and medical authors who want to add a touch of profundity to the beginning of their book chapters. Medical students and residents are steeped in Osler's aphorisms; for many of us, he is the ideal physician. There is even a large physician fan club devoted to him, the Osler Society, which holds meetings about the great man and whose members feel honored to be elected to the society. To read him is to gain insight into what young doctors are taught to aspire to become, ideals that some, at least, carry with them throughout their careers.

If some of his words resound in your mind as if delivered from the pulpit, there is a good reason for it. His father was a minister, and before he switched to medicine, Osler studied in an Anglican seminary, intending to become a clergyman himself.

The good physician treats the disease; the great physician treats the patient who has the disease.

It is much more important to know what sort of a patient has a disease than what sort of a disease a patient has.

There is no more difficult art to acquire than the art of observation, and for some men it is quite as difficult to record an observation in brief and plain language.

Listen to the patient: he is telling you the diagnosis.

The value of experience is not in seeing much, but in seeing wisely.

Medicine is a science of uncertainty and an art of probability.

We are here to add what we can to life, not to get what we can from life.

Courage and cheerfulness will not only carry you over the rough places in life, but will enable you to bring comfort and help to the weak-hearted and will console you in the sad hours.

In seeking absolute truth we aim at the unattainable and must be content with broken portions.

If you do not believe in yourself how can you expect other people to do so? If you have not an abiding faith in the profession you cannot be happy in it.

These quotations, a tiny sample of the many that circulate widely, show Osler as the enthusiastic seeker of both truth and tranquility, a man who stressed the importance of listening carefully to the patient and treating them as a person, not as a disease. He was enormously influential in molding American medical practice. He was the author of a comprehensive medical text that, although subsequently revised by others, stayed in print for a century. It was a book that became the standard for generations of students. Born a Canadian and starting his medical career there, he was one of the founding faculty members in the late nineteenth century of the new Johns Hopkins Medical School in Baltimore. This was the school Flexner used as his model of proper medical education when he did his survey of the dismal medical educational landscape.

Osler's many students (disciples, more accurately) scattered across the educational landscape to implement the vision of the great man, no doubt carrying with them little notebooks filled with his inspirational sayings. This was still true as recently as thirty years ago, when one of my colleagues did his training at Osler's old medical department; residents routinely referred to themselves as "Osler's marines," the military metaphor appropriate to how they regarded their mission of conquering the forces of medical ignorance. Osler himself later abandoned Johns Hopkins for the greater glory of England's medical establishment, ending his career as Sir William Osler, Regius Professor of Medicine at Oxford University.

Most nonphysicians regard medical training as akin to any other professional training, such as architecture or engineering. My goal in this chapter is to show you how this is not so, how all physicians are products of a system with ancient traditions and viewpoints, concepts that are impossible for doctors-in-training to avoid absorbing at least somewhat into their worldview and attitudes. Now you should understand that worldview a bit better.

In spite of all the altruistic exhortations from Osler and the others, not everything about this worldview is good, and some medical training might better be characterized as medical indoctrination. So, along with the good, you can also understand from this chapter how the long process of becoming a doctor can cause problems for physicians as we deal with patients and their families.

Regarding medicine as a special, exalted calling can help make a person a better physician, but it can also easily lead to a sense of special entitlement. Physicians sometimes take from their long educational journey an attitude that the length and arduousness of the journey itself merits special treatment, status, and consideration. The symptoms of this opinion range from assuming special parking places for our cars to expecting special deference in social and political settings that have nothing to do with medicine. Osler, and other physicians like him, were part of that trend, too. Consider this statement of his:

> The practice of medicine is an art, not a trade; a calling, not a business; a calling in which your heart will be exercised equally with your head. Often the best part of your work will have nothing to do with potions and powders, but with the exercise of an influence of the strong upon the weak, of the righteous upon the wicked, of the wise upon the foolish.

Here, in brief, he lays out what I just described; medicine is a special calling, supposedly above crass business considerations, and the physician is strong, righteous, and wise. Physicians, of course, are no more strong, righteous, or wise than anybody else. We have special knowledge and experience, as well as the privilege of tending to the sick in their time of need. That is an honor, but it is also an honor we share with many people who are not physicians.

Medical training is unusual in the way that medicine is unusual. Medicine is fundamentally an art influenced by science, a melding of modern discoveries with centuries-old observations made by doctors caring for the sick who were ignorant of what was really wrong with them. Medical training is also a twisting together of two strands—students find themselves sitting in sophisticated laboratories in the morning and following an experienced clinician in the afternoon, just as a medieval apprentice did, and learning to use examination tools that are centuries old. The marriage of these two strands, the ancient and the modern, is sometimes an uneasy one. Yet, confused and insular as it sometimes is, it is the system that produced the doctor who you may find talking to you in the hospital emergency department about your son's fever and earache. Now you know a little about how she got where she is, and that information should make it easier for you to talk to her and understand what she is saying and why.

COMMUNICATION CHECKLIST FOR PARENTS

1. Understand the tension a doctor experiences when faced with a choice of doing something and doing nothing.
2. Treatment just for the sake of doing something is rarely a good idea.
3. If the doctor appears to you a little self-important, there are deeply ingrained reasons why she might seem that way.

Chapter 8

KNOWING MORE AND MORE ABOUT LESS AND LESS

MANAGING SPECIALISTS

U nusual, complicated situations often require the special skills and knowledge of physicians who are experts in particular diseases or organ systems. The doctor initially evaluating your child may suggest consulting one of these specialists; alternatively, you may request this yourself if you think your child's problem would best be solved by involving a specialist. Some parents bring their child straight to a specialist without a referral from a more general physician. If you as a parent find yourself in either of these situations, it is very useful for you to learn about pediatric specialists—who they are, what they know, what they do not know, and how they generally practice.

Some parents make poor use of their time with specialists because they are confused over the usual role such doctors play in the care of sick children. This confusion is understandable, since the way in which medicine draws the boundaries between its various component specialties can seem bewildering. Confusion, however, can lead to poor communication, which in turn can lead to suboptimal care for your child. This chapter will tell you about these experts and how to use your time with them effectively should your child need to see one.

We should begin with some definitions. I have used the word *specialist* in the chapter title as most parents tend to use it—a doctor specializing in the care of only one organ system. However, in this chapter you will be reading about what physicians call *subspecialists*, and I will use that term from now on, because to a physician the term *specialist* means a doctor who has successfully completed one of the residency categories recognized by the American Board of Medical Specialties—internal medicine, pediatrics, obstetrics and gynecology, surgery, and so on. These doctors are certified by one of the twenty-four constituent specialty boards. So, if your child is seeing a pediatrician, she is already seeing a specialist—one specializing in the care of children. If the pediatrician thinks your child should see, for example, a pediatric cardiologist, then he is referring you to a subspecialist, in this case an expert in diseases of children's hearts.

The individual board organizations operating under the umbrella of the American Board of Medical Specialties are quite autonomous from one another and even from the overall board. The American Board of Pediatrics, for example, sets its own standards of what it means to be a pediatrician, what the training requirements are, and what material will be included on the certifying examination. Many of these autonomous boards have chosen also to establish official standards for what it means to be a certified subspecialist, what it means, for example, to be an expert in children's lung diseases or in the care of newborn infants.

For our purposes, we are interested only in subspecialties that apply to children. It is important to know, however, that not all subspecialists are supervised and certified by the Board of Pediatrics.

As you will read, some of the experts who might see your child are certified by one of several other boards, such as the Board of Surgery or the Board of Radiology. Even though these are separate entities from each other, it is fortunately true that all the boards certifying physicians who care for children generally cooperate quite closely, sometimes offering joint certification programs.

The American Board of Pediatrics was established in 1933, making it the fifth oldest of the specialty boards. It organized its first subspecialty board, pediatric cardiology, in 1961, and has since established thirteen additional subspecialty boards to certify pediatricians in a diverse range of disciplines relating to the care of children. You will read about all of these subspecialties in this chapter. But before we delve into these various fields and the circumstances in which your child might need a subspecialist, you should first understand how a doctor gets to be a subspecialist in the first place.

A physician who wants to be a pediatric subspecialist must first become a pediatrician. As you read in the last chapter, that process takes eleven years, including college, after which the prospective subspecialist enrolls in what are called fellowships. These programs are nearly always based in large children's hospitals and are approved by the supervising board to train pediatricians in the relevant subspecialty. Most fellowships last three years, at the end of which time the person is eligible to take another certifying examination; if she passes the test, she is then a board-certified subspecialist.

The process is similar for other specialties, like surgery or radiology, doctors of which also care for children at times. A surgeon or a radiologist, for example, who wants to limit her practice only to children, does a fellowship after residency in pediatric surgery or pediatric radiology, after which she takes a certifying examination.

A parent should know, however, that all these subspecialties are voluntarily designated. This means that it is not illegal for any pediatrician to declare himself a pediatric subspecialist, whether or not he has done the fellowship training and taken the test. Such "false advertising" was once quite common, especially before the widespread availability of fellowship programs. In those days, a pediatrician who had a special interest in a particular area and wished to limit his practice to this interest could simply declare himself a subspecialist in that area. Many such physicians became quite competent from either this sort of on-the-job training or by informally apprenticing themselves to acknowledged experts in the field. In fact, it was pediatricians like this who founded the subspecialties by coming together and organizing with like-minded colleagues.

These days the situation is highly structured, and all legitimate subspecialists have the proper credentials. If you wonder about the qualifications of a pediatric subspecialist who is seeing your child you can, of course, ask him. But if you are uncomfortable doing that, you can check his credentials on the Web site of the American Board of Pediatrics (http://www.abp.org); the site will tell you in what subspecialty fields the physician is certified and give the certification dates. It will also tell you if and when he recertified in the subspecialty, something now required every seven years. Many of the other boards whose diplomates care for children, such as pediatric surgery, have a similar online system for verifying certification.

Parents sometimes wonder under what circumstances a doctor will refer their child to a subspecialist and if there are any absolute rules for doing so. There are no universal standards, although parents of a child with an obvious severe heart problem, for example, will quickly find a cardiologist consulting on their child's case if one is available. There are specific procedures, such as the bronchoscopy performed on the child with the plastic toy in his airway, whose story we read in the first chapter, that only certain kinds of doctors do, and this is also a common reason for a subspecialist to enter the picture.

In general, though, an individual doctor's decision to consult a subspecialist depends upon the particular experience and knowledge base of that physician. Medicine is a broad subject, and inevitably doctors feel more confident in some aspects of their medical skills than in others. If your child's physician suggests a subspecialist, it is usually because he really does want help, and getting that help is usually best for your child. Parents can take their child to a subspecialist on their own, too, although these days many insurance plans limit the coverage they will provide if a parent does that without first getting a referral from their primary care doctor.

What follows are all the subspecialties recognized by the Board of Pediatrics, and then relevant subspecialties regulated by other specialty boards whose practitioners sometimes care for children. For each kind of subspecialist, you will learn who they are, what they do, and the likely reasons your child might need to see one of them. As you will read, most of the subspecialties listed are based upon a specific problem, but some are organized according to a child's age. Many of them parallel similar subspecialties in adults, but some do not—they are unique to children. The relationships between these various subspecialties are sometimes touchy in political ways, the doctors of each occasionally squabbling about which is the most appropriate one to care for children with this or that problem. As you read in the last chapter, a certain measure of competitiveness is something bred into physicians throughout their training. In moderation, such competitiveness is a good thing and does lead to better care for your child.

NEONATOLOGY-PERINATAL MEDICINE

The neonatal period of a child's life is birth to four weeks of age. Perinatal refers to the time just before and immediately following birth. Members of this subspecialty are called neonatologists, and they are experts in caring for newborns. Although ordinary pediatricians and family doctors also have expertise with babies and are usually the ones who care for normal newborn infants, they will consult a neonatologist if a baby is ill or has some sort of birth abnormality. By far the most common reason for a baby to need a neonatologist is if the baby is premature, born early. Such babies usually need care in a high-tech neonatal intensive care unit, which is where neonatologists spend most of their time. Although neonatologists care for all aspects of newborn infants, they often will ask their organ-based subspecialty colleagues to see an infant with a specific problem, such as a heart defect.

Most of the time a parent will not meet a neonatologist until after their child is born, when the first meeting is often in the delivery room of the hospital. However, it is increasingly common in these days of early prenatal ultrasound scanning for neonatologists to talk to expectant parents before their child is delivered if, on the basis of prenatal testing, the baby is expected to have any problems or if the mother is in premature labor and the birth of her infant cannot be stopped. As you would expect, neonatologists work closely with physician colleagues in the field of obstetrics. The obstetricians are usually the doctors who deliver the babies and care for the mother.

As a parent you might also meet a neonatologist if you bring your baby to the doctor for evaluation of some issue, for example, jaundice, and your examining doctor thinks the problem would best be handled by an expert in the field of newborn medicine.

PEDIATRIC CARDIOLOGY

Cardiologists are experts in all aspects of the heart and blood vessels. Pediatric cardiology is thus a field based upon an organ system, not the age of the child. Although cardiologists diagnose and care for children with all kinds of heart disease, by far the majority of their practice comes from the care of children with some form of congenital heart disease, one of the various malformations of the heart with which children can be born. Many of these malformations require one kind or another of heart surgery to either fix them completely or make them better, so pediatric cardiologists work closely with pediatric cardiac surgeons. It is increasingly common, though, for cardiologists to use new sophisticated and nonsurgical techniques to fix some of the less complex congenital heart problems that traditionally required an operation to correct.

Like neonatologists, cardiologists use a lot of high-tech devices. Chief among them are echocardiography machines—ultrasound instruments that allow a skilled user to diagnose most congenital heart malformations and assess how a child's heart is working. Sometimes a child needs a particularly sophisticated evaluation of his heart problem using a procedure called a cardiac catheterization. In this procedure, the cardiologist threads long monitoring devices through the child's blood vessels, typically those in the groin, up into the heart. He can then use a combination of pressure measurements and X-ray contrast studies to look at various aspects of heart structure and function. As echocardiography gets more and more sophisticated, the need for the more invasive and risky cardiac catheterization is decreasing, but many children still need the test, especially if heart surgery is planned.

The most common reason for parents to meet a cardiologist is if the doctor seeing their child wonders if the child has a heart problem. This question often arises if the doctor hears a heart murmur with her stethoscope, especially if the child has not had it before, and wonders if it is a sign of a heart problem. It is becoming increasingly common for a parent to meet a pediatric cardiologist even before her child is born. Prenatal ultrasound machines are now so sophisticated that doctors can often get a good view of the fetal heart and can sometimes identify significant heart problems in advance.

PEDIATRIC PULMONOLOGY

Pulmonology refers to the lungs, and pulmonologists are experts in diagnosing and treating all manner of pediatric lung problems. They have their own array of devices to help them do this beyond standard chest X-rays. These include bronchoscopes to look inside the lungs, CT scans to image the lungs, and mechanical ventilator machines to breathe for a child whose lungs are unable to do the job on their own. Many of the children they care for are those with serious lung conditions. A common reason you as a parent might meet a pulmonologist would be if you have a child with complicated asthma or other long-standing breathing troubles that your doctor is concerned could represent some disorder more unusual than simple pneumonia.

PEDIATRIC ENDOCRINOLOGY

The endocrine glands are the organs of the body that release hormones into the bloodstream. These include the pituitary gland in the brain, the source of many key hormones controlling a child's growth and maturation, the thyroid gland in the neck, and the reproductive glands. A large component of an endocrinologist's practice involves children with diabetes. The most common form of diabetes in childhood is caused by a complete lack of insulin, a hormone secreted by the cells in the pancreas and which regulates levels of sugar in the blood. Endocrinologists also are experts in the overall metabolism of the body—how it uses energy, makes the bones and muscles grow, and keeps the complex mixture of chemicals in the blood in normal balance.

Parents are most likely to meet a pediatric endocrinologist if their child has diabetes, is not growing or developing normally, or has a problem related to normal sexual development, such as delayed puberty. Endocrinologists are also the experts for a long list of obscure and rare metabolic disorders, so if your child's doctor is concerned about any of these possibilities, he will very likely recommend you see one.

PEDIATRIC NEPHROLOGY

Pediatric nephrologists are experts in the kidneys, as well as the rest of the urinary tract. The kidneys' main jobs are to remove body wastes from a child's bloodstream, regulate the equilibrium of the various chemicals in the blood, and maintain just the right amount of fluid in the circulation. Because nephrologists are so experienced at analyzing the balance of these things, doctors often consult them if a child's system is deranged in some way, even if the kidneys are working normally. For example, too much fluid in the system is one cause of high blood pressure, so nephrologists, along with cardiologists, are often the experts we consult about managing a child with high blood pressure.

Most pediatric nephrologists work at children's hospitals, where an important part of their practice is typically the care of children with long-term kidney failure. A key therapy for this condition is *dialysis*, the use of an artificial machine to do the work of the failing kidney. Sometimes the dialysis machine is connected to the bloodstream using large plastic tubes (*hemodialysis*) and sometimes the machine makes use of fluid introduced into the child's abdominal cavity and allowed to absorb the waste materials from the bloodstream, after which the fluid is removed (*peritoneal dialysis*). Either way, it is the nephrologist who manages this complex therapy. Most children on dialysis hope for a kidney transplant to free them from the machinery, and it is the nephrologist who cares for children before, during, and after their transplants.

Congenital malformations of the kidneys and urinary tract are not uncommon. As with the heart, prenatal ultrasound often identifies children with these abnormalities before they are even born. Most of these malformations, if diagnosed early, can be corrected, and the nephrologist plays a central role in the care of such children.

A common reason parents might meet a pediatric nephrologist would be if abnormal blood or urine tests suggest that their child's kidneys are not working normally. Besides these simple tests, nephrologists often need to order ultrasound or CT scans of the kidneys to evaluate the problem thoroughly.

PEDIATRIC HEMATOLOGY AND ONCOLOGY

This subspecialty concerns cancer and diseases of the blood. It is organized differently in children than in adult practice. In the latter, *oncology* (cancer) is separate from *hematology* (blood disorders) because most adult cancers do not involve the blood. In children, *leukemia*, or cancer of one of the blood cells, is the most common form of cancer, so hematologists, the blood experts, perform the role of diagnosing and treating all forms of childhood cancer.

Hematologists evaluate and treat all kinds of abnormalities in the blood counts, such as anemia, as well as problems in the blood clotting system, such as *hemophilia*, a genetic disorder that causes severe, prolonged bleeding. In most children's hospitals, however, it is cancer diagnosis and treatment that takes up the bulk of these doctors' practice.

The hematologist uses several kinds of tests to do her job. Fundamental is the blood count, although she will often do additional, sophisticated tests on a child's blood cells besides just counting them and sorting them into categories. Also basic to her practice is an evaluation of what is going on inside a child's bone marrow cavities, the central space in the bones where blood cells are made. To do this she places a needle into the child's marrow, usually in the hip bone, to sample what is there. (Children are normally sedated with medicine for this uncomfortable procedure.) For children with cancer of some kind, hematologists also make frequent use of CT and MRI scans to assess how their therapy is working.

Bone marrow or stem cell transplantation (which amounts to the same thing) have become important and lifesaving forms of treatment for many children with leukemia and other childhood cancers, and pediatric hematologists are the doctors who do this sophisticated kind of therapy. It is so complicated that at many children's hospitals there are hematologists who do only bone marrow transplantation.

As you can see, pediatric hematologists are subspecialists who care for children with particularly grave diseases, so it can be frightening if your doctor thinks your child needs to see one. On the other hand, if your child's doctor is concerned about an odd blood count or a question of a bleeding tendency, it is certainly best to see an expert to have those questions answered promptly and accurately.

PEDIATRIC GASTROENTEROLOGY

The gastroenterologists are the doctors who are experts on the digestive tract, the stomach and intestines, as well as the organs connected to the intestines, the liver and pancreas. Since nutrition is such an important part of pediatric practice, pediatric gastroenterologists are also the subspecialists most knowledgeable in that field.

Gastroenterologists use several specialized tests to do their evaluations. Besides blood and stool tests, these doctors make frequent use of barium contrast X-rays, ultrasounds, and CT scans of the abdominal organs. The discovery of fiber-optic technology was dramatically useful to many fields of medicine, but the gastroenterologists especially benefited from this breakthrough. They use fiberoptic endoscopes to actually see what is going on inside a child's digestive tract. They can insert these into the mouth, down to the stomach and beyond into the upper portions of the small intestine, or into the rectum and up into the large intestine. (Of course, children are sedated for these procedures.) A television screen displays what the endoscope is pointed at, giving a vivid picture of a child's insides. Gastroenterologists can do more than look through these instruments; they can also do things like remove an abnormal growth, snip off a bit of tissue for special studies, or retrieve something a child should not have eaten that is stuck in the stomach.

You might expect your child to see a gastroenterologist if your doctor is concerned about chronic or severe vomiting or diarrhea, as well as unusual abdominal pain. A child who is not growing normally might see a gastroenterologist if her doctor is concerned that she is not absorbing food properly. Abnormal blood tests of liver and pancreas function, such as you read about in chapter 4, are also common reasons for a referral to a gastroenterologist.

PEDIATRIC CRITICAL CARE MEDICINE

The previous several subspecialties you have read about were organ-centered ones, such as care of the heart, lungs, or kidneys. The subspecialty of pediatric critical care medicine is different from these; it involves the care of all a child's organs when derangements in them make a child critically ill. Like neonatologists who practice in neonatal intensive care units, critical care could be described as a geographic subspecialty, in that these doctors, called *intensivists*, generally stay in one place—the pediatric intensive care unit. They are experts in supporting all aspects of vital organ functions in children who are critically ill from a wide variety of causes.

A substantial number of children in pediatric intensive care units are there because they just had major surgery or experienced a severe injury. Many of these children have quite complicated medical and surgical problems. For children like these, the intensivist works closely with the pediatric surgeon to provide comprehensive care for all aspects of the child's situation. Intensivists also get help from many other experts. Depending upon the child's particular problem, intensivists collaborate with all the various organ-specific subspecialists. One way to describe an intensivist is as a general practitioner for the very sick child.

As a parent, you will meet an intensivist if your child is ever ill enough to need the special services available in a pediatric intensive care unit, whether the problem stems from an accident, a sickness, or a major surgical procedure. In some hospitals, pediatric intensivists also are the doctors who provide sedation to children who have procedures, such as an MRI scan or a bone marrow test, so you may meet one if your child needs a test requiring sedative medications.

PEDIATRIC ALLERGY AND IMMUNOLOGY

This subspecialty is neither organ-specific nor geographic in nature. Rather, it is system-specific. It is also organized differently from the previous subspecialties in that it has a freestanding board of its own and is not a subsidiary member of another, overarching board. The American Board of Allergy and Immunology requires those it certifies to be first either certified by the Pediatric Board (for those treating children) or the Board of Internal Medicine (for allergists who care for adults). Even though their subspecialty is not overseen by the Pediatric Board, pediatric allergists play a large role in pediatric practice because doctors frequently include the possibility of allergic problems on their differential diagnosis list for children with chronic breathing or skin problems. Asthma often has an allergic component to its symptoms, so a pediatric allergist will share the evaluation and treatment of asthmatic children with a pulmonologist—a specialist of the lungs.

Parents might meet an allergist if their child has more than mild asthma, if their doctor thinks allergies are contributing to the child's symptoms, or if the child has experienced a severe allergic reaction to something like a bee sting. Parents also may take their child to a pediatric allergist themselves if they are concerned about those things. Allergists use several kinds of blood tests, as well as skin tests and breathing tests, to do their assessment.

PEDIATRIC INFECTIOUS DISEASES

This subspecialty is distinct from the previous ones. Like critical care and neonatology, it crosses all organ systems, but unlike these subspecialties, it is concerned with the evaluation and treatment of invaders from outside a child's body—the microorganisms that cause infections. In addition, these subspecialists are the experts in developing and using vaccinations in children.

Every parent knows that children get a lot of infections. This is primarily because their immune systems are still maturing and they contract from other children a host of new viruses at day care or at school. So any doctor who cares for children is experienced in diagnosing and treating common childhood infections. Sometimes, however, a child develops an especially severe or unusual infection and needs the special expertise of a pediatrician with advanced training in that area.

The categories of problems treated by pediatric infectious disease subspecialists can be divided between severe cases of common infections and unusual infections, such as those caused by parasites and fungal microbes. Another large component of this specialist's practice is made up of children with abnormal immune systems, something that makes them unusually susceptible to severe infection. In chapter 6, you read about common antibiotic therapies we use in children; we have many, many more medications than those to treat infections, and infectious disease specialists are the experts in how to use them all.

An infectious diseases consultation is one pediatric doctors frequently request, and sometimes parents bring their children directly to these subspecialists. The usual reasons are a concern the child is having too many infections, worry that the child could have some difficult-to-find infection that is causing chronic findings like fevers, or if the child has a rare or unusual infection.

PEDIATRIC EMERGENCY MEDICINE

This subspecialty is very much like critical care in that pediatric emergency doctors work in one place, emergency departments, and care for children with all manner of organ-related problems. What these children all share is some acute problem, or change in a chronic one, that caused them to get sick enough to need evaluation in the emergency department. The subspecialty arose as it became apparent to doctors that children in these circumstances have a set of unique needs, issues best addressed by a new category of sub-specialist. Many of these doctors are also closely involved in what is called prehospital management—how ambulance and emergency transport networks work and what paramedics and first responders do for children before they reach the hospital.

Many parents meet subspecialists of this kind. In most children's hospitals, the majority of the doctors working in the emergency department are certified in the field of pediatric emergency medicine. This is presently less true in smaller hospitals or large general hospitals that care for patients of all ages. However, as the subspecialty grows, it is becoming increasingly common for most hospitals that see a significant number of children in their emergency department to hire pediatric emergency medicine subspecialists.

PEDIATRIC RHEUMATOLOGY

This is a rare subspecialty; all told, there are less than two hundred pediatric rheumatologists practicing in the entire United States. Still, most children's hospitals will have at least one, where they fill a small but important niche in caring for children. Rheumatologists are disease-specific, not organ-specific, subspecialists. They are rare because the disorders they treat, which include things like juvenile rheumatoid arthritis and lupus, are rare. These diseases share the property of causing a derangement in the child's immune system such that the body attacks itself—called *autoimmune disease.*

Your child is most likely to benefit from an evaluation from one of these experts if your doctor is concerned that an autoimmune disease may be causing the symptoms. Examples of these symptoms, which typically persist for weeks or months, are unexplained fevers, joint pain or swelling, or peculiar rashes. If your doctor recommends your child see a pediatric rheumatologist and you are not near a large children's hospital, you most likely will need to travel to such a facility to see one.

PEDIATRIC NEUROLOGY

A pediatric neurologist is certified by another cooperative kind of arrangement between subspecialty boards, in this case between the boards of neurology and pediatrics. Pediatric neurologists train first in pediatrics and then in child neurology; they are experts in all varieties of diseases and malformations that can affect a child's nervous system—the brain, spinal cord, or peripheral nerves such as those controlling pain and movement of the arms and legs.

Neurologists, as you read in chapter 3, are skilled users of the physical examination for making a diagnosis. However, they also make extensive use of brain scans, such as head CT and MRI scans. In addition, they are the doctors who read and interpret EEGs to see if a child has a seizure problem. Neurologists are the experts regarding the use of the many medications available to control seizures; if your child needs one of these medicines, most doctors will refer you to a pediatric neurologist for advice.

Your child is most likely to need a neurologist if your doctor hears something in the history or finds something on the physical examination that suggests a neurological disorder. Any seizures beyond a simple, brief one with a fever—a common thing in early childhood—merits a referral to a pediatric neurologist. Chronic headache is another common reason for a child to see a neurologist, since neurologists are the experts in diagnosing and treating migraine.

PEDIATRIC REHABILITATION

This subspecialty is devoted to diagnosing and treating patients with physical disabilities of many kinds. Its practitioners, known as *physiatrists*, are certified by their own specialty board. Those who wish to be certified as pediatric rehabilitation experts take additional training, usually at a children's hospital.

Children who benefit from this kind of expertise are those who have a congenital malformation of their bones or nervous system that interferes with normal functioning, or who suffer some disease or injury that leads to such a problem. Physiatrists are often quite involved in the rehabilitation of sports injuries, so this is a common reason for a referral to such a doctor. Physiatrists often work on a team of doctors from other subspecialties, such as orthopedic surgeons and neurologists, as well as physical therapists, who together provide multidisciplinary care for children.

DEVELOPMENTAL AND BEHAVIORAL PEDIATRICS

This subspecialty, a component of the Board of Pediatrics, consists of pediatricians specially trained in the developmental and behavioral aspects of children's health. The subspecialty board arose to fill an evolving need for doctors who were particularly interested in and knowledgeable about those aspects of pediatric practice that did not involve acute illness, injury, or an organ-related problem. Over the past decades, more and more of pediatric practice has involved questions of normal development and behavior, especially in office practice. The increasing diagnosis among children of attention deficit hyperactivity disorder, and the therapies prescribed for this condition, is just one example of this trend. These subspecialists are finding themselves more and more in demand.

You as a parent are most likely to meet a developmental specialist if you or your doctor are concerned that something your child is doing, or not doing, is not normal. If there is some kind of abnormal behavior, subspecialists of this kind can tell you exactly why and what you should do about it, if anything. These *develop-*

mentalists are especially interested in all aspects of a child's environment, such as home and school settings, and how these affect the child.

ADOLESCENT MEDICINE

The subspecialty of adolescent medicine, like neonatology, is organized according to the age of the child, although on the opposite end of the childhood age spectrum. Unlike neonatology, however, it is decidedly low-tech, and adolescent subspecialists primarily see their patients in an outpatient rather than hospital setting. Adolescence is a special time of life; people of that age may have the physiology of adults, with their bodies mostly grown up, but may not have many of the other characteristics of adults. It can be hard to convince adolescents to see the doctor. They almost never want to sit in a waiting room filled with fussy young children, and many pediatricians do see mostly infants and preschool children. Family medicine doctors also typically see a large number of babies and small children. Adolescent specialists bridge the gap between pediatric "baby doctors" and the internal medicine doctors who care for adults. As a parent, if there is an adolescent pediatric subspecialist available, you may find that your child would much rather see a doctor like that.

PEDIATRIC SURGERY

Children not only have unique medical needs; they have special surgical ones, too. Pediatric surgery is a subspecialty of the American Board of Surgery, and surgeons who wish to become pediatric surgeons must first train as general surgeons, after which they do a fellowship in pediatric surgery. All children's hospitals have pediatric surgeons, and many medium- and smaller-sized facilities that care for children do as well.

Although general surgeons—those who operate on adults—are usually fully competent to perform straightforward procedures on older children, the younger the child, the more he needs the special expertise of a pediatric surgeon. This is most true for infants, especially premature infants. If your doctor asks a surgeon to see your child—for abdominal pain, for example—it is fair to ask if the surgeon is a pediatric one, and, if not, how experienced the surgeon is in operating on children.

PEDIATRIC ORTHOPEDIC SURGERY

Orthopedic surgery concerns the diagnosis and treatment of disorders of the bones and joints. Orthopedists also traditionally take care of many muscular and soft tissue problems in the arms and legs. They often care for sports injuries, and many orthopedists are deeply involved in the practice of sports medicine, in which they collaborate closely with physiatrists and physical therapists.

Subspecialists who practice pediatric orthopedics are closely analogous to pediatric surgeons in their training. A doctor wishing to become a pediatric orthopedist must first do a residency in orthopedic surgery, then a fellowship in pediatric orthopedics, typically at a children's hospital.

Children have a large number of unique issues regarding their growing bones. In addition, there are many kinds of congenital abnormalities of the bones and joints that can affect children. Pediatric orthopedists are experts in diagnosing and managing all of these, including those that do not require surgery.

Active children break a lot of bones, so the most common

reason you might see a pediatric orthopedist is if your child breaks a bone. General orthopedic surgeons, those not specially trained in pediatrics, are fully capable of treating many broken bones in children, particularly older children. However, there are many situations that call for the expertise of a pediatric orthopedist, such as certain kinds of broken bones and problems with bone growth. As a parent, it is best to ask your doctor for a referral to a pediatric orthopedist if one is available. If there is not an available specialist nearby, and your child's problem is not an acute one like a broken bone, it may be advisable to travel to see a specialist.

PEDIATRIC UROLOGY

As with orthopedics, other aspects of surgical practice are divided along anatomical lines. A urologist is a surgeon trained to operate on the kidneys and urinary tract. This field has its own board, the Board of Urology, a body that offers special advanced certification for urologists who complete a fellowship in pediatric urology.

Similar to the situation with pediatric surgery and pediatric orthopedics, all urologists are trained to operate on older, larger children, particularly if the operation is for a condition children share with adults. Pediatric urologists are most important for conditions peculiar to very young children, particularly congenital malformations of the urinary tract. Some of these conditions require extensive reconstructive surgery and are best done by a urologist with that specific training and certification. If your child has such a condition, a pediatric urologist is the best person to handle it.

PEDIATRIC OTOLARYNGOLOGY

This is another anatomy-based surgical specialty, often abbreviated ENT for ear, nose, and throat. It has its own governing specialty board. If your child needs surgical expertise in one of these parts of the body, the situation is similar to a child who needs a subspecialist in urology or orthopedics, also organ- or body-specific subspecialties. All ENT surgeons are trained to perform common pediatric procedures such as taking out the tonsils and adenoids or placing pressure-equalization tubes in a child's ears for chronic ear infections. Pediatric ENT surgeons, who have additional training and certification, are most important if your child needs extensive surgery in one of these areas at a very young age.

PEDIATRIC OPHTHALMOLOGY

An *ophthalmologist* is a physician who is trained in diagnosing and treating diseases of the eye, including performing surgery on the eye. Often parents confuse ophthalmologists with *optometrists*, who are not physicians. The latter perform eye examinations and fit glasses, and in some states have privileges to treat certain kinds of eye diseases. Some of the eye problems children can have are similar to adult disorders, and a nonpediatric eye specialist is fine for those situations, but children also can have eye problems adults do not have, and pediatric ophthalmologists have advanced training to diagnose and treat them. If your child has one of these special eye disorders, it is a good idea to see if a trained pediatric ophthalmologist is available in your area. If not, and depending upon the complexity of the specific problem, it is worth considering traveling to consult one.

CHILD AND ADOLESCENT PSYCHIATRY

This subspecialty describes a psychiatrist who has advanced training and certification in diagnosing and treating mental health problems in children. A prospective child and adolescent psychiatrist trains first as a psychiatrist and then does a fellowship in the subspecialty; she is thus not required to be a pediatrician first, although many do begin or even complete training as pediatricians before their interest in child psychiatry induces them to move on to that field. Any parent of an adolescent can attest to the unique psyches of adolescents. For that reason, although many general psychiatrists do some pediatric practice, it is usually best for parents to seek out a child and adolescent subspecialist if their child needs psychiatric care.

Often parents are confused about the difference between a psychologist and a psychiatrist. It is easy to see why they would be confused, because, besides the similar names, what some kinds of psychologists do and what psychiatrists do often overlap, and the two kinds of mental health professionals often cooperate with each other, which can be helpful to the child but also can confuse the issue further. In brief, a psychologist is usually a doctor but not a physician—she typically holds a PhD degree, not an MD. The treatment modalities the two types use are often similar. However, as a physician, a psychiatrist is licensed to prescribe any medications the child needs; in contrast, a psychologist generally uses treatment approaches that do not involve medicines, although some states allow limited prescribing by psychologists of selected medicines.

What a parent should know about this complicated web of how various mental health professionals practice is that each community is different, and you should not be ruled by the specific categories of providers. If your child needs the expertise of practitioners like this, you should investigate the situation in your area and learn about who your child's doctor recommends as an appropriate person to help your child get the care she needs.

ϒ   ϒ   ϒ

We have now learned about all the basic kinds of subspecialists who take care of children. It is a long menu indeed. If your doctor wants to refer your child to one of these doctors, or if you want to seek one out on your own, there are some important general things you should know beforehand about subspecialists and how they operate. Over the years, I have found that many parents assume pediatric subspecialists are akin to smarter versions of general pediatricians; after all, they have twice as much training treating children as do generalists. Shouldn't they know more than ordinary pediatricians? The answer is: sometimes, but often not.

Subspecialists nearly always have different perspectives on children's problems than do pediatricians or family doctors; sometimes this is helpful, sometimes less than helpful, but it often means they do not share the same medical viewpoint of more general physicians. I write this as a subspecialist myself with over two decades of experience dealing with other subspecialists. If you are to communicate effectively with people like me, you should learn about how and why we are different.

This chapter's title is "knowing more and more about less and less." This is not my own expression. The phrase is a common, usually good-natured jibe generalists toss at subspecialists, and, like many of the sayings listed in the previous chapter, there is a good measure of truth in the observation. Subspecialists do indeed know a great deal about their chosen field, but this knowledge comes at a cost—we tend to ignore aspects of pediatric practice that have little to do with our subspecialty.

I have met the occasional subspecialist who truly is a brilliant polymath, someone well-versed in her own field but still as knowl-edgeable about the broad area of pediatrics as most generalists. Such people are rare, though. Perhaps this is because the new things we learn crowd out what we already know. Arthur Conan Doyle, in his first Sherlock Holmes story, famously put forth his theory of how the brain works—that it has only a fixed total capacity for retaining knowledge. Holmes accordingly took pains not to learn anything of no use to his detective work; Doctor Watson was aston-ished to discover that Holmes was ignorant of the fact that the earth revolved around the sun. Experts in brain physiology would prob-ably disagree with the fictional detective—we can always learn new things without forgetting old ones—but all would agree we tend to forget things we once knew well but have used little lately. This sit-uation describes many subspecialists.

All pediatric subspecialists in those disciplines regulated by the American Board of Pediatrics are board-certified pediatricians, meaning they once went through all the training and took all the tests to qualify as pediatric generalists. Some future subspecialists even practice general pediatrics for a time until their interests or circum-stances lead them to enroll in a subspecialty fellowship. Physicians like that have made some use of their broad-based skills in the past and so tend to remember them longer than those subspecialists who went directly from residency training into fellowship without ever doing general work. Even so, many subspecialists in practice today have not practiced general pediatrics in decades, if ever. Inevitably, they have missed some important developments that have occurred outside their narrow interest, in the broader field of children's healthcare.

The Pediatric Board is well aware of this tendency of subspe-cialists who do little outside their particular niche to forget what they once knew. The board regards it as a potential problem and has addressed the problem in several ways. All certifications, whether of subspecialists or of general pediatricians, are now time-limited at seven years, after which the doctor must recertify. The recertification process is more than just taking another test; the physician must also show evidence of keeping up with the field by reading and going to educational meetings.

Time-limiting the board certificates ensures that any subspecialist your child sees is current in her knowledge base. The board went even further, however; now subspecialists must also keep current their certification in general pediatrics if they want to stay certified in their subspecialties. This is to ensure that pediatric subspecialists do not become rusty in their general pediatric knowledge base.

In spite of these efforts by the board, as pediatric subspecialists know more and more about less and less, they are bound to know progressively less and less about more and more: less about all the things outside their range of expertise. The longer they practice their subspecialty exclusively, the greater this effect. So if your child is being evaluated by a subspecialist with decades of experience in her field, the good news is that she is probably a very capable subspecialist; the bad news, however, is that she is unlikely to know about the latest in pediatric care outside her field. In addition, there are still a large number of subspecialists who received their certificates before the new time-limited requirements took effect. Many of these have lifetime certifications for their general pediatric boards and are never required to update their broader skill set.

Why does this matter to parents? It matters because you cannot be assured that the subspecialist will take into account all aspects of your child's medical situation, particularly those that fall outside her area of expertise. Sometimes a general pediatrician consults a subspecialist with a fairly open-ended request, something like "I'm confused about what's wrong with this child, but I think you can help—can you?" At other times, the pediatrician spells out quite explicitly what question he wants the subspecialist to answer, such as: "Does this child have a heart problem?"

In the first sort of request, the generalist is asking the subspecialist for any ideas she might have; in the second, he is making a specific request of her. The answer he gets thus depends upon the question he asked. It also depends upon the personality and practice style of the particular subspecialist. Some subspecialists, no matter the original request, dive into the child's problem and ponder along with the generalist what the cause might be, even if it is outside the subspecialist's bailiwick. That is often helpful, although remember the caveats about how knowledgeable subspecialists may or may not be regarding things beyond their usual scope of practice.

Some subspecialists, as a matter of course, confine their answer to what is asked of them. For example, her answer to the question "Does this child have a heart problem?" could simply be "No." That is helpful as far as it goes, but if the doctor sent your child to the cardiologist because he wondered if the chest pain or shortness of breath was caused by the heart, he is still left with the issue of how to explain the symptoms.

Subspecialists who are themselves pediatricians, even if their general skills are a little creaky, are more likely than nonpediatricians to offer general advice outside their own particular niche if they think they can help explain your child's problem. Subspecialists who are not pediatricians more typically answer the narrower question. For example, a pediatric orthopedist treating the issue of whether your child's limp is caused by a bone and joint problem is likely to stick to answering that question. Or an adolescent psychiatrist, if asked whether a child's headache is caused by depression, may just reply that it is not. These kinds of answers, important as they are, may be all you get out of a subspecialist.

Subspecialty consultations can be crucially important for getting your child's health needs taken care of, but, as you can see, using them wisely requires a certain amount of filtering of their answers. Your child's general pediatrician or family doctor is the ideal person to do this. If you decide to bring your child to see a subspecialist without a referral, realize you will need to be the one who relates what the doctor tells you to the larger picture of your child's health. This may not be an issue if the problem is clear-cut—a broken wrist, for example. But it may be a problem if your child's complaint is more vague—wrist pain, for example. Realize also that insurance plans vary in the degree to which they will cover visits to a subspecialist without a preexisting referral. If you do wish to take your child on your own, you should check with your insurance carrier about that.

You can see how involving subspecialists in a child's care can require parents to be even more involved in coordinating things. This is especially so if more than one subspecialist is seeing the child. The situation is analogous to one you read about in chapter 4: how sometimes too many laboratory tests, especially those ordered in a scattershot way, can be more confusing than enlightening. Sometimes a child with an unusually complicated or obscure problem is evaluated by two, three, or even more subspecialists. Sometimes these doctors disagree with one another, occasionally quite strongly, about what to do.

These disagreements can have significant consequences if the bone of contention is something like, for example, the need for a major operation or a risky test. As you have read, doctors are not known for having small egos, and once in a while parents get caught in the middle of the squabbling among doctors. When I have seen that happen, all concerned truly believed they were advocating in the best interests of the child. The question is: who is best qualified to decide what those best interests are?

The answer is: you, the parent. If you find yourself in that uncomfortable situation, the best help comes from your child's general pediatrician or family doctor—a doctor who knows your child well and can look at the entire picture dispassionately. And fundamentally, parents make excellent choices for their children. I have seen and been involved with many such controversial cases over the years, and in every case the parents, uninformed as they may be of medical science, made the best decision. We should not be surprised by that; after all, it is the parents who know their child the best.

COMMUNICATION CHECKLIST FOR PARENTS

1. If your doctor suggests your child should see a subspecialist, ask specifically what question or questions the expert will be expected to answer.
2. If you think your child should see a subspecialist, it is best to ask your doctor about it and get a referral; your insurance plan may require this, and your doctor will have the best insight regarding which subspecialist to consult.
3. After your child has seen the subspecialist, discuss the findings and recommendations with your regular doctor.
4. Neither you nor your doctor is obligated to take the advice of the subspecialist expert, whose viewpoint may be narrower than yours.
5. If you wish to research the qualifications of a subspecialist, the American Board of Medical Specialties (http://www.abms.org) can guide you to the individual specialty board for that doctor. For pediatricians, you will find a subspecialist's qualifications at the American Board of Pediatrics (http://www.abp.org).

Chapter 9
WHEN THE CONVERSATION TURNS SOUR

HOW TO HANDLE A DIFFICULT DOCTOR

My goal throughout this book has been to give you insight into how physicians think—how we conceptualize, evaluate, and solve children's clinical problems. My model has been one of a conversation, a two-way exchange in which both parents and doctors do their best to understand the viewpoint of each other and together reach a satisfactory outcome—diagnosing and treating the child.

Sometimes, however, this ideal situation does not occur, and the conversation fails. One cause for potential failure is mutual incomprehension of each other, a situation often exacerbated by the pressured atmosphere of the emergency department or walk-in clinic. This is especially so for complicated situations; it often seems there is far too little time for the detailed medical history these children require. From the doctor's standpoint, another cause can be difficult parents who seem either unwilling or unable to provide a coherent medical history. Sometimes, though, the cause is not difficult parents; it is a difficult doctor.

237

There are, of course, varying degrees of such difficulties. Individuals have individual personalities, and it is inevitable that some parents will not mesh well with some doctors. Difficult encounters may be less than optimal, but they can still result in a good outcome for the child. Most parents would choose to get on well with their child's doctor if possible, but, if that does not happen, they certainly want the doctor to be correct in his diagnosis and treatment. Personality clashes are less important during one-time encounters— situations where the family will most likely never see that doctor again. Such clashes matter most when dealing with a physician in a long-term relationship.

What happens when communication between parents and doctors misfires and the fault lies with the physician? If your appointment with this doctor was for some long-standing problem, you can certainly choose to make a subsequent appointment with another physician, with little lost except for time. It is different for acute problems. Unfortunately, these situations do not leave parents with many options. After all, if you have waited several hours in a crowded waiting room to see the doctor you are unlikely to demand to see another one, assuming one is available, because you are not communicating well with the first one; you are more likely to do the best you can for your child with the one you have.

Physicians can be difficult from a parent's perspective for many reasons. Doctors working in a chaotic emergency department may have the added stress of juggling the problems of several sick children simultaneously. Other reasons may stem from the doctor's personal circumstances; for example, perhaps he has a headache, a sore back, or has just gotten a disturbing telephone call from his son's school principal. Sometimes, however, the explanation is just the pure cussedness of the doctor. Medicine is a healing profession, but the reality is that not everyone in it is a saint, or even a pleasant person.

It should come as no surprise to parents that the doctor they find difficult to deal with is often a problem for his colleagues as well. And, as is true for parents, a doctor dealing with a contrary fellow physician often has limited options regarding what to do about it. Here is a common example of what I mean. If your child needs to visit the emergency department in the middle of the night and the physician there telephones an on-call subspecialist to ask for advice, only to have that subspecialist berate her for bothering him at such a late hour, this inter-physician encounter is unlikely to go well. Thus we doctors occasionally face the same kinds of inter-personal communication problems parents have with doctors. Unlike parents, however, our insider viewpoint gives us some tools to deal with the problem.

Before we delve into some of the specific ways parents may find doctors difficult, you should think about one issue I have found causes particular discomfort for many parents—their perceived need to be reasonable and nice. I certainly am not advising anyone to be unduly rude or unpleasant. But it seems to me that parents, in an effort to be nice, sometimes tolerate fairly obnoxious behavior by physicians more than they should. Hard as it may be, you really should not care what the doctor thinks of you. It is not your job to be nice; your job is to be the best advocate you can for your child. This may sound harsh, but it is true. Fortunately, most doctors, like most parents, are reasonable people, so this issue does not arise too often. This chapter will help you in those hopefully rare instances when you must deal with a difficult doctor.

We begin with a general survey of the more common ways I have noted over the years that physicians can be difficult for parents to deal with. Several of these categories and specific situations are interrelated, and most are not unique to medicine; anyone who works in a wide spectrum of occupations requiring close interpersonal relations has likely met representative examples of such people already.

I also begin this section with a confession: I have no doubt been guilty at various times and in varying degrees of committing all these sins myself. Sometimes I realized it at the time, sometimes I needed others—nurses, physician colleagues, even parents—to point it out to me. Sometimes, like anyone, I was surprised people had thought my demeanor was a problem. It was especially at those times that I needed to be told about it and, at least in retrospect, appreciated that someone had done so.

THE POOR CONVERSATIONALIST

A key theme of this book has been how the ideal encounter between a physician and the parents of an ill child is a conversation among *equals*. The doctor knows more about medicine, but the parents know more about their child. Each party applies their own expertise toward solving the child's problem. Some physicians, for one reason or another, are not good conversationalists in this sense.

There are several common versions of the poor medical conversationalist; all of them have corresponding parallels in nonmedical settings. Often the most basic difficulty is one of manner. A good conversationalist is a person who, no matter what he is thinking, clearly shows interest in what the other person is saying. The doctor who from the outset acts distracted, hurried, or even uninterested gets the conversation very much off on the wrong foot, especially if parents have been waiting a long time to see her. This sort of doctor may avoid eye contact with you or may continually write while you speak. Although most of us take notes during an interview, parents not unreasonably expect us to look up at them now and then.

A poor conversationalist is impatient to get at what she assumes to be the crux of the matter and will interrupt parents, cutting off their explanations. It is true that the doctor typically directs the flow of conversation, but she needs to do this in a way that does not stifle it. If she is too heavy-handed, the result is a very one-sided conversational exchange, which can in turn result in suboptimal medical care for the child. As you read in the chapter about the medical history, knowing how to guide and direct rambling historians is a delicate skill for physicians, and we all learn to do this to some extent. The poor conversationalist, however, often errs on the side of demanding from parents short, even yes or no answers only, to the questions she asks. She does not want all the details. Like Officer Friday on "Dragnet," she wants "just the facts, ma'am."

Besides being annoying, the doctor who is a poor conversationalist will miss things, occasionally important things, because there are times when it is the details that really matter. A doctor like this often glances at the child or the chart and makes a snap judgment about which way to go with the interview when it has barely begun. Already convinced about what is important, she may interrupt parents who she perceives as wandering from the key points of the history. She also may end the history before the parents have said all they want to say, thereby missing crucial bits of information.

Even though we physicians in clinical practice spend a good portion of our day talking to people, many of us still have bad conversational habits—mannerisms, speaking styles—that impede communication. Some medical school curricula have lately begun to include systematic instruction in how to speak during patient encounters, but most of us picked up how to do this as best we could from listening to and watching our bedside teachers. This makes for uneven history-taking skills among physicians.

Our innate personal conversational styles can also interfere with the process. This may cause little problem in other aspects of our lives, but it can interfere with our roles as physicians. Some of us mumble, others of us gaze at the ceiling when talking, and still others use convoluted ways of expressing ourselves. Some of us present ourselves as amiable conversationalists, others come across to parents as unduly grumpy. If you find yourself trying to understand what a soft-spoken, mumbling doctor with an irritating facial tic is trying to say to you, remind yourself that this person may well be an excellent physician for your child, exasperating as it is for you to understand what he is saying to you.

Parents who find themselves opposite a physician who is a poor conversationalist for any of these or many other reasons often become frustrated, and sometimes angry. After all, you have been waiting to see this person, sometimes for hours, or you may have made this evaluation appointment for your child weeks in advance. Now your concern is to get the most for your child out of an interview that seems to be moving in an unsatisfactory direction: how can you do this?

I think the most crucial thing is to remind yourself that you and the doctor truly are partners in the diagnostic and therapeutic enterprise, and most doctors, no matter how harried and frazzled at the moment, realize and understand this if given the chance. If you, as a parent and as a partner with the doctor, feel the interview is going seriously offtrack, there are concrete things you can do to restore its direction. You can do this because you now know how medical history taking works. Use that knowledge to show the doctor you understand how she frames the problem in her mind.

For example, show that you know how important it is to present your child's symptoms in the order they occurred, what they were associated with, and what made them better or worse. Be as precise as possible. Remember to stick to one symptom or complaint at a time. A doctor who is already a marginal conversationalist often becomes an interrupting, controlling interviewer if she perceives that a parent is aimlessly wandering around with disjointed answers to her questions. Once an interview goes seriously awry in that way, it is very difficult to restore the situation.

Another useful approach is to ask the doctor what things are on her differential diagnosis; she may list things for which there are key points in your child's history you had not thought to mention. A good time to do this is when the doctor is doing her physical examination; even the most dominating interviewer will usually relax her control while she is examining your child, allowing you to revisit anything in the history that concerns you. If you do take that approach, however, remember the obvious point of not asking questions at inopportune moments, such as when the doctor has a stethoscope in her ears.

THE POOR EXPLAINER

A physician, like anyone, can be a poor explainer of things for several reasons. Some of these reasons are common roadblocks to good communication between parents and doctors. Foremost among these is the tendency to use medical jargon. This is not a problem unique to doctors. When I take my car in for repairs, I often must ask the mechanic to explain what is wrong in a way I can understand. I have a rudimentary understanding of what the various parts of the engine do, and I even recognize the terms he uses to describe these parts, but I have little understanding of how the parts relate to each other and what can go wrong with them. Automobile mechanics often wrongly assume that most people know more than they actually do about car engines. If you spend all day working with engines and talking with colleagues who are doing the same thing, it can be difficult to grasp how confusing the subject can be to nonmechanics.

Physicians find themselves in an analogous situation. Most parents know about their child's body and many of the ailments that can affect it in the same way I know about my car and what can go wrong with it. But even though we know the words for body or engine parts, someone explaining to us what is wrong with a child or a car should not mistake this passing acquaintance with the vocabulary as true understanding—explanations should be in plain, jargon-free English.

There is another way this situation is analogous to auto mechanics: often the nonmechanically inclined, especially men, believe they *ought* to know about car engines, even if they do not, and are reluctant to press for clearer explanations from the mechanic. So they nod wisely while the mechanic explains, all the while having little or no idea what he is talking about. Likewise parents sometimes feel as if not being medically knowledgeable makes them somehow poorer parents, and they are reluctant to press the doctor for clearer explanations when they do not understand what she is telling them. You should not let your mechanic do anything to your car you do not understand the need for; do not accept any less from your child's doctor.

There are some physicians who are poor explainers of things not because they use jargon but because they are just plain poor explainers of anything, medical or otherwise. This is uncommon, though, since most of us do spend such a large part of our time talking and explaining that eventually we become better at it just from constant practice. These days, a more common issue is language: when the native languages of the parents and the doctor are not the same and one or both parties is struggling with expressing themselves in clear English. Since medicine is in many ways a universal language, physicians who are not native English-speakers may have a particular tendency to use medical jargon more than they should because that is the idiom they know best.

What should parents do if they find themselves with a doctor who is a poor explainer, either from her excessive use of medical jargon or some other reason? I think the best approach is to do as a doctor does when we take a history from parents who are vague and imprecise in their descriptions: we pause frequently and rephrase our questions in different ways, and keep doing that until we understand. Parents can do the same thing by stopping the conversation at intervals, restating in their own words what they think they are hearing, and then asking the doctor if that is correct. Thus a parent can respond to a murky explanation from the doctor with something like: "So, what I hear you saying is _____. Is that right?"

The worst thing for your sick child is to imply to the doctor you understand when you do not. One way or another, make her explain it to you so you understand it. Make her draw pictures if necessary. When you insist on continuing the conversation until you comprehend everything, you are not being a pest, you are doing your job of being a good parent.

THE NONEXPLAINER

How doctors treat patients' need for information has changed significantly over the past few decades. Sixty years ago, medical practice was much more paternalistic than it is now, although some would say it continues to be so in important ways. Still, not too long ago it was common for doctors to tell patients or their families next to nothing about what was going on. The presumption always was: the doctor knows best. It was felt that telling patients and families the truth, accurately explaining the ins and outs of what was happening in a way they could understand, placed an unreasonable psychological burden on them; only the doctor had the strength of character to bear this burden.

Physicians no longer espouse that viewpoint. These days we maintain, or ought to, that patients are the ones who control their care. This does not mean that patients call all the shots and select all aspects of what the doctor will do, but it does mean that patients are in charge of important decisions affecting their bodies. For children, this means parents make the key choices.

It is the doctor's obligation to explain to you, in a way you can understand, what is wrong with your child and what he proposes to do about it. Sometimes parents feel as if they are imposing on the doctor, inappropriately taking up his time, when they ask him to convince them he is evaluating their child in the best way. This is decidedly not the case; however, a doctor who is a nonexplainer can make parents feel this way by either resisting their questions or by implying that he is doing them a courtesy by answering them. He is not doing them a favor; answering their questions is part of his job.

Parents whose child is being evaluated by a nonexplaining physician should simply press him for answers until they are satisfied. There is generally no need for confrontation. In fact, I have observed physicians who are chronic nonexplainers actually think they explain things satisfactorily and are genuinely surprised when told they do not. In most instances, the nonexplaining doctor is simply a variety of the poorly explaining doctor.

There are some physicians who do a reasonably good job explaining what they think is the problem but who for some reason resist telling parents the details about the tests they are ordering. Such doctors often say something to the parents like "We'll check some tests," and then leave it at that. But as you learned in chapter 4, parents are the ones who will be doing the lion's share of the actual explaining to their children about what is happening, so parents need to know explicit details about what is going to happen. Any parent who has dealt with the constant "Mommy, why?" of a five-year-old knows this well. So ask about those tests, particularly if they involve anything painful or frightening for your child.

THE DISBELIEVER

All good doctors learn to filter what parents say to them during history taking, to examine each parental statement for reliability, likelihood, and sheer outlandishness. Parents of sick children are a cross-section of humanity and, like all of us, vary in their observational skills, their ability to express themselves, and their tendency to exaggerate or minimize what they see. Parents, not being physicians, may not notice and comment on things a doctor would notice. Good doctors also understand that parents of sick children, especially very sick children, are stressed by their situation and sometimes rendered more than a little incoherent by that.

In spite of all these issues, the fundamental principle of medical interviewing is that parents are virtually always telling the truth as they understand it. They will not see things as through a doctor's eyes (unless they have read this book, of course), but they will nearly always faithfully report what they see if the doctor is reasonably skillful at bringing out the salient points during the conversation. Unless a doctor has very compelling evidence to the contrary, she assumes goodwill on the part of the parents. What that means in practice is that parents who give disorganized, difficult-to-interpret histories are not intentionally trying to deceive her; they are simply doing the best they can to describe what they see. The disbelieving doctor is not inclined to trust the truth of that statement.

This variety of poorly communicating doctor can be a troublesome one for parents to deal with. She may seem pleasant in conversation, but this kind of doctor also may come across to parents as brusque, even antagonistic and confrontational in demeanor. Parents interviewed by doctors like this sometimes feel as if they are being cross-examined, not interviewed; instead of a two-way, mutual conversation, the encounter feels more like a grilling by a suspicious police officer. That is an extreme description, but it is

one parents have used when telling me about unsatisfactory encounters with doctors. Milder metaphors I have heard from parents
about these situations include feeling like a teenager being quizzed
by a parent over staying out too late, or like a student who has mis-
laid his homework assignment.

There are several underlying themes for this kind of dysfunc-
tional conversation. One is that parents feel as if the doctor does not
really believe what they are saying, as if the parents need to produce some objective evidence to prove that what they are saying is
true. The nuance can be subtle, but nonetheless obvious. If most
doctors hear a parent say, "Johnny had a fever," they will follow up
by asking how high the fever was. If the parent's reply is something
like "I didn't take it—he felt hot," most doctors note that fact and
proceed with the interview. In contrast, the disbelieving doctor is
inclined to say something like "Why didn't you take his temperature?" or "Why don't you have a thermometer?"

Physicians inclined to disbelieve what parents say to them are,
at root, manifesting the old tendency for physicians to set themselves above the patient. Treating what parents have to say as being
at best uninformed, at worst outright deceptive, is another example
of how some doctors regard themselves as superior to others. It is
another face of medical paternalism. From what I have seen over
the years, I suspect that this attitude and behavior is a little more
prevalent in pediatric practice than in other kinds of medical
encounters because many parents of infants and young children are,
in comparison to the doctor, themselves young. An age disparity
between parents young enough to be a middle-aged doctor's children and the doctor can make the doctor behave a little like a parent
herself in how she treats her patient's parents.

What should parents do if they find themselves meeting this
kind of doctor? My best advice is to realize they are unlikely to
change the doctor's behavior much, and that overt confrontation

generally does not work well because it tends to confirm in the disbelieving doctor's mind her impression that parents, rather than being allies in the child's evaluation process, are more often unreliable adversaries. It works better for parents to recognize what is happening and respond by taking extra pains to be precise and consistent in what they say, perhaps using statements like "This may seem strange to you, but . . ." or "I know I should have paid more attention to the rash, but it seemed to me at the time that . . ."

An extreme tendency to disbelieve what parents are saying is a bad trait in a physician, and it likely will impede her ability to do the best job for the child. But as with other kinds of poor physician communicators, I think most disbelieving physicians are not fully aware of how their manner interferes with their interactions with parents. Still, it is not a parent's job to educate the doctor about that, and it is probably best not to try.

THE POOR LISTENER

This type of physician deserves its own category, although in some ways it represents a blend between the poor conversationalist whose mannerisms get in the way of good communication and the disbeliever who hears what parents are saying but does not believe it, and thus could be said to be hardly listening. Another version of the poorly listening physician is one who is not listening with an open mind or open ears because he has already formulated a diagnosis. He tends to search through what parents are saying for points that fit the problem into a preconceived diagnostic box. This sort of doctor is ignoring that bit of sage advice from William Osler: "Listen to the patient—he is telling you the diagnosis."

Parents should be careful, however, about assuming that the doctor is not listening to what they are saying. As you read in the chapter about history taking, doctors are trained to ask the same questions more than once, especially if the answers are crucial to the diagnosis. This repetition ensures that you understand what he is asking and also allows the doctor to approach your child's problem from several directions and thereby identify all the key details. An experienced doctor often anticipates parents' worry that he is not listening by saying things like "I know I've asked you this already, but I want to be clear about . . ."

There is a variant of the poorly listening doctor that I have encountered from time to time. This is the doctor who asks parents if they have any questions about what is happening with their child but then does not answer them; instead, he answers other, often related questions, perhaps those he thought the parents should have asked but did not. If you find yourself in this situation, it is best simply to ask your questions again until you are satisfied with the answers. Doctors of this sort typically will take as much time as necessary to answer your questions; they just may need a bit of role reversal, with you, the parent, asking the same question several different ways as doctors do when taking a history.

THE DISPARAGER

Doctors who disparage, or even ridicule, what parents tell them are, fortunately, rare. Nevertheless, sometimes parents may infer from what the doctor says or how he acts that he does not value what they are telling him, even though he did not mean to imply such a thing. All physicians have had the experience of overly touchy parents inappropriately assuming from our questions that we do not respect their ability to give a useful answer. This is prone to happen in situations where parents, already agitated over their child's illness, are concerned that the doctor believes at least part of their child's problem stems from what the parents did or did not do. A good, experienced physician easily senses this defensiveness in parents and does or says things to reassure them; the disparaging physician does not bother, since he assumes parents are usually part of the problem anyway.

Doctors with this kind of poor communication skill overlap those who are disbelievers, since both place little stock in what parents are telling them. The disparager is a little different from the disbeliever, however. Whereas the latter may actually be contemptuous of parents' ability to give a good history, the former usually carries in his manner some of the old medical paternalism; the doctor knows best, and the parents know very little that is helpful, but that is not their fault—they cannot help themselves.

Parents may meet a doctor with this attitude, although, truth to tell, such a physician is more often identified out of parental earshot, since most have the good sense and manners not to act in an obviously disparaging way toward parents. These doctors generally confine their comments to colleagues or nursing staff, although they are occasionally surprised by how good parents' hearing is through a partly open examining room door.

What should you do if you meet such a doctor? Unfortunately, and as with the related category of the disbelieving physician, you as a parent can do little to change this doctor's personality type. You can, however, be aware of what is happening with the interpersonal dynamics of the medical interview. This insight should be all you need to understand that the doctor's disparaging manner is not about you, the parent; it is about him, the doctor, and he probably behaves in a similar way to many other parents and patients. Try not to take it personally. Besides, as long as his medical skills are up to the task, he is still probably a good source to give the care your child needs.

You will not be surprised to learn that doctors who are disparaging toward parents are also often disparaging toward their medical and nursing colleagues. This can make parents uncomfortable as when, for example, a doctor who is seeing their child criticizes what other doctors have said or done. It is one thing to be honest and open with parents; doctors should not conceal from them things they have a right to know. But it is quite another thing to denigrate one's professional peers. Doctors who habitually do this often seem to do so in order to make themselves look more important in parents' eyes. You should be wary of participating in such a conversation.

THE JUDGE

I have placed this kind of doctor in her own category, although the poor communication traits one finds among physicians like this do overlap some of the others, especially the disbeliever and the disparager. I have done this because the conversational barrier one finds between parents and judging physicians is somewhat different from the other two.

All physicians naturally make judgments regarding the parents they are interviewing. For example, we assess how accurate and plausible their history is. We try to decide if they are telling us the whole story and, if not, if they are inadvertently or deliberately holding something back from us for whatever reason. All experienced physicians do this; what we rarely do is judge the parents' worth as people, as individuals apart from their children. There are exceptions to this, like all blanket statements in medicine, but we cannot do a good job abiding by the important ethical principle of equal care for all children if we categorize parents as good or bad. After all, children do not choose their parents.

The inappropriately judging physician runs the risk of allowing her opinion of a child's parents to get in the way of her taking proper care of the child. Her judgments might be condemning or laudatory; either type can cause problems because they lead to assumptions that may not be correct. Physicians should be especially vigilant about the dangers of inappropriate judging when there are social differences between them and parents, such as ethnicity or language. All humans have the capacity to be good parents. I have seen convicted felons who are better parents in comparison to people who are social pillars of their communities.

Interestingly, judging physicians sometimes err by overvaluing the position of the parents. One sees this occasionally when one or both parents are medical professionals. There is a real risk for miscommunication if the evaluating doctor assumes that parents' medical or nursing knowledge means they are perfect observers and historians. When their children are ill, parents who are doctors or nurses are parents first and need to be treated that way.

Unfortunately, there is not much advice I can offer if you believe that a physician's judgment of you as a person is interfering with her assessment and management of your child's medical problems. As with other potential communication problems between parents and doctors, confrontation is rarely a good strategy, since a physician guilty of this communication problem is unlikely to admit it or even recognize it. My best advice is, armed with what you have learned in the previous chapters, to do the best you can to ensure that your child's evaluation—the history, physical examination, and laboratory tests—is as thorough as it needs to be, and that the doctor, whatever you think of her, explains things completely.

THE EGOTIST

Egotism is a common and unflattering trait among doctors, although most of us keep it under adequate control when dealing with patients. Throughout this book, the ideal doctor-parent encounter has been described as a collaboration among equals, each of which brings expertise to the exchange; the doctor knows medicine, the parent knows the child. This is the ideal, although sometimes the reality falls short of it. The way our medical system is now structured gives more power and influence to the doctor side of the relationship than the patient side. As you read in chapter 7, things were not always this way; a century ago a surplus of doctors with treatments of doubtful usefulness scrambled to attract patients. These days, however, physicians have many more therapies that actually work, plus the benefit of an enormous medical establishment behind them. So now doctors are usually the ones deciding who gets what treatment. In spite of that fact, good, experienced doctors will do their best to use their power over patients lightly, always inviting parents and patients to share in the authority.

Physician egotism can get in the way of good communication in several ways. A simple manifestation is the tug-of-war over whose time is more valuable, the doctor's or the parents'. A good example of this conflict is the doctor who schedules far more patient appointments than he can accommodate in a day, then seems unaware of how keeping a parent waiting for hours can poison the atmosphere even before the evaluation has begun. Parents usually understand long waits when they take their child to the doctor for an unanticipated acute problem. If the waiting room is full of children just like theirs, there is little the doctor can do except see them each in turn. But the subspecialist who packs his waiting room with too many scheduled patients is proclaiming, in effect, that his time is far more valuable than that of parents, who often must take off a full day's work to bring their child to see him.

The egotistical doctor is one who tends to forget that the patient is the center of everything, the reason the parents are there in the first place. He forgets that the encounter is about the child, not the doctor. This attitude can show itself in a persistent tendency to turn the subject of the conversation away from the child and toward the doctor. The result may be harmless, as when a garrulous doctor is genuinely trying to relax the parents and their child with a friendly conversation about other things, or it may be more toxic, as when a doctor constantly talks about himself and what he does. The latter can be particularly trying to parents who have waited a long time to see the doctor, only to find their brief time with him taken up by extraneous chatter.

Although it can be annoying to parents, excessive egotism in your child's doctor is generally a minor issue in the big picture of getting your child the evaluation she needs. I say this because, although there are exceptions to everything, for the large majority of doctors I have met who are more egotistical than the average, their self-centeredness does not get in the way of their medical skills. In fact, some subspecialties, such as high-risk surgery, almost require the physician to have a huge ego if he is to perform such surgeries effectively.

So it is largely a matter of the personal taste of the parents. If you find yourself irritated when talking with an excessively egotistical doctor, and if you think this is interfering with his proper evaluation of your child, the best thing to do is to be persistent in turning the conversation back to your child at every opportunity. Of course, if you are really irritated by his manner or the way he treats you, do your best not to see him again.

THE DEFENSIVE

I divide this kind of communication blocker into two varieties: physician personality and physician mode of practice. The physician with a defensive personality is one who interprets questions from parents as questioning of her medical judgment. Unlike the supremely egotistical doctor, who is often sufficiently secure in his image of himself that he is magnanimous toward parents who ask questions, the overly defensive physician has the opposite sort of personality; she may be inwardly or outwardly unsure of herself and often responds to parental questions in self-justifying ways that can border on the argumentative. Parents easily sense this attitude. For example, I have heard exchanges in which the parent feels a need to begin a question to the doctor with something like "I'm not questioning your medical judgment, but what about . . ."

Physicians with naturally defensive personalities probably had those tendencies reinforced in their medical training, since students and residents are often closely questioned, even roughly attacked, by superiors who believe this sort of hazing is a vital part of teaching young doctors. These kinds of teachers are becoming rarer, but there are still enough of them out there that students who fall into their clutches emerge from the experience with whatever defensive tendencies they already had greatly enhanced. Rather than welcoming parents' questions as an important tool for two-way communication, they are more likely to feel threatened when a parent asks them probing or even quite innocent questions.

A bigger potential problem for parents with sick children is not the physician with a defensive personality but the physician who practices defensively. You read in chapter 4 how medical testing, excessively and inappropriately used, can cause major problems and even place a child at significant risk. Physicians who practice defensively usually order too many tests, thinking that by doing so they are both helping the child and covering their own backsides. In fact, poorly justified, "shotgun" lab testing does neither of these things. Much has been written about how physicians defensively order too many tests because they worry about being sued for malpractice if they miss something. This may be true to some extent.

However, my own observation is that physicians who practice this way would probably do so even if the threat of malpractice litigation did not exist, since defensive medical practice is to a great extent a function of the physician's personality.

Doctors who are excessively defensive in their use of medical tests also tend to use subspecialty consultations in the same way. Very sick children with complicated problems often need the knowledge and skills of experts. But as a subspecialist myself, I know that some doctors call in the subspecialists largely to spread the responsibility more than anything else, a behavior we call "loading the boat." You read in the last chapter how to make effective use of subspecialists should your child need one. If you find an overly defensive doctor evaluating your child, you may also find that you need to take an active role in questioning the appropriateness of consulting subspecialists. And remember—subspecialists often want even more tests and procedures, potentially adding still more unneeded complexity to your child's situation.

THE AVOIDER

Most of us are, to some degree, procrastinators. We avoid or postpone doing unpleasant things. In this sense, physicians who are avoiders are no different from anyone else. For a doctor, however, avoiding things often leads to poor, or at least less than frank, communication with parents.

One kind of avoidance behavior is when the doctor avoids answering your questions. These doctors do not behave this way because they are poor listeners; they just find it uncomfortable to answer your questions. Often this doctor takes the oblique approach of not quite answering the question you asked, and instead rephrasing it into a question he would rather answer. He tends to talk around issues, especially those that are part of serious, unpleasant, or intractable medical problems. He also tends to use euphemisms for unpleasant things, commonly retreating into medical jargon because medical language seems more sanitized and neutral.

I have considerable professional experience with avoiders because my own subspecialty of critical care often presents parents and physicians with difficult choices, situations in which there are sometimes no good options, just less bad ones. Many times I have spoken with parents who, after an interview with a physician who is an avoider, must ask me what the doctor really meant to say. And that is the key to the avoiding-type of physician: he probably thinks he is doing what is best by filtering what he says and not speaking directly, but parents invariably want their questions answered as directly as possible. If you find yourself in an interview with a doctor like this, you really have no option except to press him for an explicit answer to the question you actually asked, not the one he chose to answer.

There is one other variety of the avoiding physician encountered by parents whose child has ongoing medical problems. This is the doctor who just plain avoids them and their child. These are doctors who only reluctantly return your telephone calls or, if your child is admitted to the hospital, always seem to miss you when they come around to see your child in her room. This seems like odd behavior for a physician, but it is not rare. The reason for it is that the doctor procrastinates or even avoids conversations that he believes, for any number of reasons, will be difficult or uncomfortable either for you or for him. Of course, that is all the more reason to have the discussion. Nothing interferes more with a conversation than one of the parties not showing up to partake in it.

THE POOR EXAMINER

It sounds difficult to believe, but some doctors are simply not good examiners of children. I do not mean that they were not properly trained or that they are incompetent; they simply are not smooth when performing an exam. You will virtually never find this quality in pediatricians or exclusively pediatric subspecialists, but you will occasionally meet physicians whose scope of practice spans the pediatric age spectrum but who are much more proficient in examining older patients than they are dealing with children.

Sometimes this problem is largely a social one; every parent knows it takes a special knack to put a toddler, older child, or adolescent at ease during a physical examination. Each of these developmental stages has its own particular nuances, and facility in examining children from infancy to young adulthood is something some doctors never really master. Even though a doctor's examination may be effective in that she correctly identifies the problem, she may still make the child or the parents uncomfortable with how she does it.

If you and your child are dealing with a physician like this, your new knowledge of how doctors routinely examine children can help the situation. You can reassure your child about what is going on and what comes next, something the doctor ought to do but may forget, given her particular communication problem. You can help the doctor position your child for the examination, such as for a toddler's ear check or a school-age child's abdominal examination. In my experience, most physicians of this sort appreciate such parental assistance very much because they fully realize examining children, especially uncooperative children, is not their strong suit.

֎   ֎   ֎

I do not wish to leave you with the impression that I think most doctors cannot communicate with parents. Most doctors are good at it, although all have their own personal styles. Practicing anything makes one better, and doctors who care for children spend much of their day talking to parents. Medicine also offers students several levels of self-selection, and those who find themselves to be poor or uncomfortable communicators often choose a medical field in which their lack of those skills does not matter so much. Parents should know that the doctor they are dealing with chose to do what he is doing; he is talking to you because he enjoys conversational encounters like the one he is having with you. You may feel, in the particular moment you meet him, that this is not obvious, but fundamentally he is talking to you and your child because he likes it. You should be reassured by that fact.

There remain those rare times when friction, for whatever reason, between parents and doctors causes the situation to explode in a way beyond rescuing. Unfortunate as these events are, the several I have seen had one overriding cause: poor or complete lack of communication between parents and doctors from the very beginning of the encounter. The poor communication led to misunderstandings, the misunderstandings led to mistrust, the mistrust led to increasingly acrimonious accusations, and the final result for at least one of the parties was the hasty arrival of a hospital security guard to restore order. No one wants that; it is the sick child who ultimately pays the price for the adults' inability to get along.

But what should you do if you are concerned or even angry over how a doctor is dealing with you? It is a difficult thing for most parents to confront the doctor on the spot, and doing so is usually counterproductive for their child's needs. Besides that, many parents are intimidated by the doctor's authority—the traditional deference we usually give to someone in a long, white coat with a stethoscope around his neck is a powerful thing—and they are reluctant to press the issue.

If you find yourself in such an unfortunate and unpleasant situation during a routine office visit, the solution is easy—complete the visit and do not go back to that doctor. But if it happens in a large facility, such as a hospital emergency department, it is best for you, for your child, for other children, and for the hospital that you tell someone about it. Nearly all hospitals have a mechanism for doing this, often through someone who carries a title like "patient representative." The idea is to have an impartial third party, one over whom the doctor has no authority, hear your story. This person may not be available on the spot at the time of your visit, but it is easy to find out how to contact them—ask the nurses or call the hospital administration department. The doctor needs to know about what happened from your perspective, and the patient representative is the one to mediate.

Ultimately it does not matter who is "right" in failed doctor-patient encounters; it is sufficient that you, the parent, believe you were poorly served. Both the doctor and the hospital also need to know that. Doctors who are poor communicators usually exhibit a long-standing pattern of annoying and frustrating their patients' parents and, odd as it sounds, they may be oblivious of this behavior. Somebody needs to tell them. The parents and children that doctor sees in the future will be in your debt.

This chapter on dealing with difficult doctors and poor communicators brings us to a close in our discussion on how to talk to the doctor. You have read how pediatric physicians are trained, how we evaluate sick children, how we decide what to do with sick children, and a little about our personality quirks—in short, how we think. In this final chapter, I will do my best to put you, the parent, beside me—even inside my head, as I lay out a series of clinical cases. You can try your hand at thinking as my colleagues and I think and solving these diagnostic puzzles as we would solve them.

COMMUNICATION CHECKLIST FOR PARENTS

1. If you do not understand the doctor, or if you do not think the doctor has understood you, the time to intervene is as it happens, not later.
2. It is both the doctor's job and responsibility to communicate with you in a way you understand; you are not imposing on him if you insist on this.
3. If you believe a doctor's behavior has been inappropriate, you should strongly consider contacting the institution's patient representative to express your concerns.

Chapter 10
PUTTING IT ALL TOGETHER
Solving Problems as a Doctor Does

The previous chapters have described how doctors listen to you as parents and examine your child, how we determine what tests to order and what to do with the results, how we combine these components and use them to diagnose what is wrong with your child, and finally how we decide what to do for your child. You have read about how to help your child's doctor as he works his way through these various steps, principally by learning how to talk to him in a manner he will understand and how to listen to and interpret what he is saying. Our last chapter brings the whole process together by inviting you, the parent, to join me as I evaluate a series of real-life examples, taken from children I have actually cared for myself. Some are simple, some are far from simple.

CASE ONE

I take a chart folder from the box at the door of an examining room in the emergency department. Stapled to the front of the folder is a one-page form, at the top of which the nurse has written: "four-year-old with two days of cough and fever," followed by the vital signs of oral temperature (101.4), heart rate (96 beats per minute), respiratory rate (32 breaths per minute), and oxygen saturations (95 percent, which indicates a normal amount of oxygen in the blood). Thus before even beginning the evaluation, I see that the boy has more than a history of fever; he has a documented abnormal temperature of greater than 101 degrees. The temperature is not dangerously high, though, so I do not expect the child to look critically ill. His respiratory rate is also mildly elevated. So even before opening the door—though mindful of the need not to prejudge the case too much—I anticipate finding a child with some respiratory problem that is giving him a fever.

As I come through the door, I hear the child cough several times. It is a dry cough; I do not hear the sound of mucus rattling in his throat, and the cough comes in three to six bursts. The child is sitting in his mother's lap. He looks a bit anxious, but he seems alert as he looks at a picture book with his mother.

Thus before I have said anything at all I am forming a tentative differential diagnosis list in my mind. At the top is respiratory infection—upper respiratory at least, and, because of the rapid breathing rate, possibly pneumonia. I remind myself again not to jump to a diagnosis too fast—he could have fever and cough from one or more of several other causes—but "common things are common."

As I talk to the mother, I find out several key things in the child's history. He was fine until three days ago, when his symptoms began with fever. The cough began the next day and has steadily worsened. He was not able to sleep last night because whenever he lies down, his cough gets worse. The mother gave him some over-the-counter cough medicine, but it did not help. She has given him Tylenol for his fever, and although it brings his temperature down, the fever comes back several hours later. He has never had anything like this before and has no other medical problems. His appetite has decreased with the illness, but he has been eating and drinking some. He has an older brother with mild asthma. No one else at home is sick, but several children at his school are out with respiratory ailments.

This is the history I hear from the mother. I am sure that, with what you have learned thus far, you can yourself frame the questions I asked in order to get the history, particularly the chief complaint, the history of present illness, the past medical history, the social history, and the systems review. Also notice that the history the mother gave me is slightly different from the one she gave the nurse; she told me the fever began three days ago, a day before the cough started. As you have read, that sort of omission is typical. Often parents remember things between the time they talk with the nurse and then with the doctor; this is why we always ask the same questions more than once. Even though some parents find this a little irritating, it is important for the doctor to do because it often uncovers more information about the child's condition.

I begin my exam by letting the child stay sitting in his mother's lap. This is a useful trick to use for an anxious child; one can usually examine the head, ears, throat, neck, and chest of a cooperative four-year-old this way, and he is more likely to stay cooperative if I let him stay in his mother's lap. He will need to lie down for a good abdominal examination, however.

I look into his ears with my otoscope; the drums are a little red but generally look normal. Since he is four, I ask him if his ears hurt, and he answers no. I feel his neck gently and find that he has a few mildly enlarged glands under his jaw. I need to look in his throat, but that will probably upset him a little (or a lot)—most four-year-olds already know about that uncomfortable throat stick doctors use to depress the tongue. So I skip ahead in the standard order of the examination to listen to his chest with my stethoscope because I want to assess his heart and lungs while he is still cooperative.

Before I listen, though, I watch him breathe. I also notice he is still coughing in the same pattern every few minutes. The nurse has already replaced his shirt with a hospital gown, so I lift that up to have a look. I glance at the clock on the wall as he breathes, counting the breaths in fifteen seconds; I count eight, which, multiplied by four, verifies the nurse's measurement of mildly increased breathing rate. Even though he is breathing a little too fast, I do not see any sign of increased work of breathing—no retractions under his ribs or at the top of his breastbone. As I watch, I wrap my hand around the end of my stethoscope to warm it up because my goal, when I press it against his chest, is to listen to his breathing while he is comfortable and quiet. Nothing makes a child jump more than placing an ice-cold stethoscope on his bare chest.

I listen to the back of his chest first. This allows him to turn his face and body toward the comfort of his mother. In addition, a doctor can usually hear signs of pneumonia best at the lower aspect of the lungs in the middle of the back on either side of the spine. Once I have listened to a few quiet breaths, I ask him to take several deep breaths, showing him what I mean. The effort makes him cough, but in between coughs I hear a few crackles on the left side. I cannot be sure of the right side because he is getting a little restless; as a practical matter, however, once I have heard crackles on one side, it does not matter much if I do not get a good assessment of the other side. Now he is getting more upset, and it is hard for me to get a good listen to the front of his chest, which is why I examined his back first—that is where the money is in hunting for signs of pneumonia.

At this point in the evaluation, I am leaning more and more toward a diagnosis of pneumonia. This child has fever, cough, rapid breathing, and crackles in the chest. There is little else this could be besides pneumonia. I do need to decide what kind of pneumonia it is, even though doing so is mostly an inexact calculation of probabilities. I also need to complete my examination. You have read about how important it is to be thorough, and it is a mistake to stop at this point because one never knows what else will show itself. In this case I have his mother lay him down on the cot and get a quick look at the back of his throat; it is a little red back there, but his tonsils look normal. His abdomen is normal, as is the rest of his examination. A pertinent negative finding is that he has no rash.

So this child certainly has pneumonia, but I should try to see how extensive it is, even though his normal oxygen saturation and normal work of breathing suggest it is not too severe. The best way to assess things is with a chest X-ray, so I order one. What about blood tests—does he need any of those?

If the child looked more ill, if he showed increased respiratory effort beyond the mild increase in breathing rate, or if his mother told me he had not been drinking much, I would probably get a complete blood count and an electrolyte panel. I would also probably get a blood culture to see if he has bacteria in his bloodstream. This is very much a judgment call based on physician experience, but for this child I would stop with the chest X-ray. Some doctors might not even do that if the crackles make the diagnosis of pneumonia quite obvious. He does not look dehydrated to me and does not look like he will need intravenous fluids; if he did look that way, I would definitely get the blood tests.

I send the child off for his chest X-ray, which shows evidence of mild to moderate pneumonia in both lungs. Antibiotics help bacterial pneumonia but do nothing for viral pneumonia, but since there is no way for me to tell the difference, I give the mother a prescription for an oral antibiotic and send them home after making arrangements for the child to see his regular doctor the next day for a check on how he is doing. If the child had looked sicker, had low oxygen saturation values, or had a worse X-ray, I would have strongly considered admitting him to the hospital for intravenous antibiotics and oxygen. This case was milder, so home he went. In sum, this case represented a common thing behaving in the common way.

CASE TWO

My next case evaluation also takes place in the emergency department. This child is a bit sicker than the last one. In fact, the nurse jumped him ahead in the line of those waiting to be seen because she was more worried about him. Pulling the chart from the wall slot, I read the brief description: "ten-year-old with fever, headache, and sore neck for one day." The child's vital signs show a temperature of 104 degrees and a rapid pulse but a normal respiratory rate. These are concerning symptoms.

When I open the examining room door I see the boy lying on his side on the cot. His mother sits beside him. The room is a little dim because his mother turned down the lights when he complained they hurt his eyes. Now I am even more concerned, because *photophobia*, a condition indicated by painful sensitivity to light, is one of the classic symptoms of meningitis—infection around the brain. So is a stiff neck.

The mother tells me that her son has been sick since the day before, when he first complained of a headache and wanted only to lie down in his room. His mother took his temperature and found he had a fever, for which she gave him ibuprofen (Motrin, Advil); this helped both the fever and the headache. He then ate dinner but vomited afterward. The mother checked on him several times during the night; he still had a dull headache and a mild fever, for which she gave him more ibuprofen. The next day he was not better and had the new complaint of a sore neck, so she brought him to the hospital. He had eaten nothing and drunk very little during the past eight hours.

After hearing this story, I am even more concerned. In fact, as I listen to the mother I am starting my physical examination, because meningitis is a serious disease that needs immediate treatment. Meanwhile, she tells me a few more things about him. He is generally healthy but does have occasional migraine headaches, usually triggered by overexertion and fatigue. He just returned from a weeklong session of summer camp the day before he became ill; the mother did not know if other children at the camp were sick. All of these details could fit with meningitis, so that is uppermost in my mind, at the top of my differential diagnosis list.

As I examine him, however, I uncover a few other things. For one thing, he is quite alert in spite of his headache, which is a pounding one, and able to talk to me. He tells me it hurts to swallow. When I look into his mouth, I see that his throat is a little red; his tonsils are normal-appearing, but the back of his throat is red.

He also tells me more about the neck pain. The neck pain of meningitis is in the back of the neck. It is caused by spasm of the neck muscles, making it hurt to flex the neck forward and touch the chin to the chest. This child's neck pain is not like that. What is bothering him is the front of his neck. I find out why when I gently feel the area under his jaw and down the front of his neck; he has a chain of several glands on either side of his voice box that feel enlarged and are tender when I touch them. He will not flex his neck forward because it hurts too much, however, so I am still concerned about meningitis.

Continuing my examination, I see he has a fine rash of tiny, reddish bumps across his chest and upper arms. The bumps feel like sandpaper when I rub my fingers across them. The rash does not hurt or itch and looks more red along the inner lines of his elbows. When I examine his abdomen, he complains of mild, diffuse tenderness when I push on it, but nothing localized to one place, like the right lower quadrant where the appendix is.

My differential diagnosis list has now expanded to several items. Meningitis is still at the top because it is such a serious infection and missing it is potentially life-threatening. It is more than just important for me to weigh this possibility against other diagnoses; it is vital that I actively search for reasons this child does *not* have meningitis—I need to positively rule it out. So meningitis stays on the list. But what about the sore throat, rash, and abdominal pain? Could those be signs of meningitis, too?

Infection from some of the microorganisms that cause meningitis can cause a rash, although not usually one that looks quite like this child's rash. This rash, plus the sore, reddish throat and the swollen glands in the front of his neck lead me to put something else on the differential diagnosis list—strep throat. Although many children with strep throat will have an impressively red throat with enlarged tonsils, not all of them do. Headache and mild abdominal pain are also common with strep infection in school-age children, and he has just spent the past week in close quarters with a busload of his contemporaries.

My diagnostic dilemma is a common one faced by doctors in the emergency department. I have several items on my list, bacterial meningitis and strep infection, followed by viral sore throat plus a migraine headache. The last of these could explain the vomiting and photophobia, and his mother told me his usual migraine triggers are fatigue and overexertion, two things this child most likely experienced after a week at summer camp. The headache also sounds more like migraine than meningitis. What should I do now?

The first thing I do is explain my dilemma to the child's mother. Statistically, the most likely thing he has is strep. When I mention this to the mother, she suddenly recalls (recollections like this are often triggered by new information) that he has had several strep infections in the past, all of which gave him a headache. Yet even though strep throat is the most likely problem, the possibility of meningitis, though far less likely, has very serious implications. The upshot is that I need to do some tests.

Since I need to get some blood tests (the old standbys of complete blood count, differential count, and serum electrolyte panel) and the child looks a little dehydrated to me, with dry, cracked lips and tongue, I start an intravenous line in his hand, get the blood for the tests, and give him an intravenous salt solution to fix the dehydration. Once the fluid is in, he says his head feels better, too. I swab the back of his throat with a cotton-tipped applicator to get a rapid strep test, which most of the time tells me within an hour or two if it is strep.

The blood counts come back showing an elevated white blood cell count, which suggests a bacterial infection, as does the abnormal shift in the differential count. His blood chemistries verify that he was dehydrated and needed the intravenous fluid. The throat swab for strep is not back yet, which is not unusual. Should I pursue the possibility of meningitis further? His headache is better—perhaps it was just a migraine, not a brain infection.

I am still pondering whether to do a spinal tap on this child. It is the only way to positively rule out the possibility of meningitis, but the procedure can be painful and frightening to the child, so I do not want to do it needlessly. On the other hand, we doctors *want* most spinal taps to show no evidence of infection; if every tap is positive, then we are not doing enough of them and are missing some cases of meningitis. I go back to reassess the child; he says the light still hurts his eyes, and now it does seem to me that his neck hurts not only in the front but is also a little stiff in the back. He also seems more lethargic than he was an hour ago, maybe even a little confused, another sign of potential meningitis. That is enough for me—I discuss with the mother the need for a spinal tap, and she agrees.

But what about the strep test? Should I wait until it comes back from the laboratory? If it is positive for strep, then does the child still need the tap? The answer, in spite of Occam's razor and my reluctance to "give" the child two diseases, is that he still needs the tap because he could have both things. In fact, strep can even cause meningitis, although this is very rare.

So, after explaining everything to the mother, I do the spinal tap. For this procedure, I can give the child some sedative and pain-killing medicines through his intravenous line to minimize the discomfort. When all the tests come back from the laboratory, the results show a positive throat culture for strep and a normal spinal fluid examination—no meningitis. I give the child penicillin for his strep, give a little more fluid in his veins, and then send him home with a prescription for more penicillin and instructions to see his regular doctor the next day if he is not better.

This case demonstrates a typical diagnostic problem, one that turned out to be an uncommon presentation (headache, photophobia, rash) of a common thing (strep throat). Also typical in this story is what doctors do when we have a serious item on our differential diagnosis list, something we do not want to miss but that is not the most likely diagnosis.

CASE THREE

The next child comes with her mother to the emergency department one weekend afternoon. I sigh a little when I take the chart from the door rack and read the chief complaint: "fourteen-year-old girl with abdominal pain and vomiting off and on for months." The reason for my initial annoyance is that the emergency department is not a good setting to evaluate a child with months and months of symptoms, especially intermittent ones. Emergency departments and walk-in clinics are not set up to solve long-standing problems; they are designed to solve acute issues, with the emphasis on getting the children seen and then either back out the door or, if they are too sick to go home, up to a bed in the hospital. If you bring your child to such a facility for an intermittent, chronic symptom, you stand a good chance of leaving frustrated and unsatisfied.

However, there are perfectly good reasons for a parent to bring their child to the emergency department for a chronic problem. For example, a child may be experiencing an exacerbation of a problem that cannot wait for an appointment with his regular doctor—worsening asthma, for example. Or a child may develop a new, worrisome symptom that his parent is concerned may be connected with his chronic problem, such as a newly noticed fast heart rate in a child with a known heart problem. The key point in these examples, however—something that distinguishes them in a visit to an acute-care facility for long-standing symptoms—is that the former group of parents are visiting the emergency department for a focused answer to a specific question.

In spite of the general inadvisability of bringing their child to the emergency department on a Sunday afternoon for vague symptoms, parents still do this on occasion. One common reason is their dissatisfaction or frustration with the inability of previous doctors to figure out what was wrong with their child. Another is that the child's symptoms have been only intermittent and may not have been present when a previous doctor saw the child; many parents have had the frustration of making an appointment to see the doctor for something that, when the appointment time finally arrives, is no longer there. Depending upon the symptom—abdominal pain, for example—the doctor sometimes tells the parents to come back when the symptoms recur. If that is a weekend afternoon, then usually the only place available is the emergency department.

If you as a parent find yourself in this situation, realize that the doctor will most likely be a stranger who will undoubtedly cringe a little as I did when he reads the words "off and on for months," followed by "seen several doctors already without a diagnosis." So it is a good idea to be especially prepared with the clear and succinct history you now know how to give the doctor.

Returning to our case at hand, as I enter the room I see the child lying on the cot reading a book while her mother sits beside her scribbling notes on a pad. The mother looks up; the child keeps reading. I try to look as encouraging as I can, but already I wonder about how this interview will go. The mother is ready for me, meeting my unspoken concern head-on. She tells me she knows this is not the best way to do things, but she has been so frustrated with previous doctor visits that she feels desperate about getting some kind of answer about her daughter's chronic abdominal pain.

She tells me her daughter's pain has been going on for several months at least, possibly longer; it is hard to tell because the girl does not always admit to having any discomfort. The pain seems to be made worse by eating, and the child has vomited occasionally, although this has not been consistent. Since this is an adolescent, old enough to help with the history, I turn to the girl to ask her about the pain. She puts down her book and seems willing to cooperate.

She describes the pain as a cramping sort of pain, coming in waves that last a couple of minutes before subsiding. Most of the time the pain is in the lower right part of her abdomen, although sometimes it is more diffuse across her belly. The overall episodes of worsening and improvement usually span a couple of days; one of these began last night, although she feels little discomfort at the moment. The girl confirms her mother's statement that the pain is often worse an hour or so after meals. She gives the additional information that often a bowel movement makes it feel better, and that she has had some occasional diarrhea. Several times she has seen blood in her stool, most recently yesterday. I ask both of them about fever, rash, or any other associated symptoms when the periods of pain come; neither can recall anything.

As we talk, I am forming my tentative differential diagnosis list in my head. There are several categories of disorders that come into a doctor's head when he hears a story like this. Chronic intestinal infection is one of them, something that can be caused by several kinds of bacteria or even parasites, particularly one called *Giardia lamblia*. I ask about travel and about the family's living environment; they went to Mexico last year (a common source of intestinal infections for American tourists who may not be as careful as they should be with drinking water), but that was long before the symptoms began. They live in town and drink city water. The child has not been exposed to farm animals, another potential source.

Since the child's symptoms seem to be worse after meals, I next ask if she or her mother have noticed any associations with specific foods. The mother has thought about that question a lot, and had initially assumed that food intolerance was the cause. She had read up on the long list of maladies that are caused by what we call malabsorption syndromes, symptoms caused by an inability of the intestines to digest a particular food, and had already tried, in a commendably systematic way, to cut these specific things, especially sugars and wheat products, from her daughter's diet to see if such elimination diets helped. None did.

Any pain in the right lower quadrant of the abdomen always makes us think of appendicitis. The most common variety is acute appendicitis, the rapid progression of the peritoneal signs—the sharp, severe pain that is worse when the abdomen is jiggled in any way—which you read about in chapter 3—that tell us it is time to call a surgeon. Sometimes, though, the appendix can become chronically inflamed and can even rupture, then seal itself off again. This can lead to a very serious situation, and it can also cause the sort of intermittent symptoms this child is having, so I am adding this possibility to my mental list.

I next ask the mother what previous doctors had thought about the problem. She answers by bringing up another item that belongs on every differential diagnosis list for children with intermittent abdominal pain—the so-called functional pain you read about in the chapter on history taking. This term describes pain for which the doctor can find no physical cause. It is often related to various kinds of stress and is a very common cause—probably the most common—for chronic mild pain in children.

The mother had taken her daughter twice to the doctor. On both occasions, he told the mother he believed the pain was functional, but his evaluation was handicapped by the fact that the child was not having any pain when he examined her. He did not do any tests, but he did tell the mother to take her child to a doctor when she was having the pain—hence today's inconvenient Sunday visit to the emergency department. He also told her to keep track of when the pain occurred (only on school days, for example) and what made it better or worse, which was why this mother was so well prepared to give an excellent history.

As our conversation continues through all the elements of the history, we reach the systems review portion of the interview. I have already noticed that the girl looks small for a fourteen-year-old and has little outward sign of maturation—no breast development, no acne at all on her face. I ask about that, a question that, when dealing with girls, is best approached by asking about her menstrual periods. They tell me she has not had her first period yet. This is not necessarily abnormal, but it is unusual. The average age for a girl's first period in this country is twelve years old, two years younger than this girl's age.

The history completed, I move on to the physical examination. I still have all the items I discussed previously on my nascent differential diagnosis list, but I have moved functional pain toward the bottom, primarily because of what appears to be the girl's delayed growth and her history of occasional diarrhea with blood in it; the latter of these in particular is not consistent with a functional explanation. (In fairness to the first doctor, the child had not noticed this symptom at the time he evaluated her.) When I examine the child, I find her abdomen to be mildly tender in her right lower region and I feel a suggestion, just a vague hint, that she has an abnormal fullness in that area, possibly a mass about the size of a small lemon. Now I know what tests to order.

Putting together everything as a doctor does, I have deduced that this girl has a several-month history of intermittent abdominal pain, sometimes accompanied by vomiting and bloody diarrhea, and what feels like a tender lump in the lower right quadrant of her abdomen. She is not acutely ill at this time and has no fever. She has had markedly delayed growth. She may have a chronically inflamed or perforated appendix, but I am more concerned about the possibility of what we call inflammatory bowel disease, particularly a disorder called Crohn's disease. The growth failure in particular is highly characteristic of this disease.

This differential diagnosis list guides the tests I need to order. She needs the standard blood counts and blood chemistries, plus a liver panel and something we call the sedimentation rate, an exquisitely sensitive indicator of inflammation going on somewhere in the body. She also needs an abdominal ultrasound or CT scan to define what that lump is. Since I am going to ask a surgeon to consult on the case, I wait to see which imaging modality she prefers; she wants the CT scan, so I order that.

The results of these tests show that the child most likely has Crohn's disease, not an appendiceal abscess. The tenderness was an area of local inflammation of her intestine. The practical question for that Sunday afternoon is answered: the child has no condition that needs an immediate operation. She does, however, need to see a pediatric gastroenterologist. They are the experts in managing Crohn's disease, and *managing* is the best term in this case because the disorder lasts a lifetime, although with treatment most children can live nearly normal lives. I arrange for her to see a specialist the next day.

So in this case, we actually made a complicated diagnosis not of a common condition, such as functional abdominal pain or infectious diarrhea, and not of a common condition presenting in an uncommon way, such as chronic appendicitis, but of a very uncommon disorder. (Crohn's disease has a prevalence of about fifty cases in every one hundred thousand persons.) And we did it in the emergency department on a busy Sunday afternoon. What made this possible? It happened because the child had a well-informed mother who had thought long and hard about what was wrong and had organized her thoughts extremely well. She thought like a doctor does.

CASE FOUR

The next case begins in the emergency department, too. As with the previous case, I notice immediately on the child's chart that the nurse recorded the fact that the child had been ill for several weeks at least. The reason he is here now, though, looks to be a potentially serious new problem. The chart reads: "Twelve-year-old boy with several weeks of cough and fever; seen several doctors without a diagnosis; this morning started to cough up blood." The nurse recorded vital signs indicating a low-grade fever and mild elevation of heart rate.

As soon as I open the examining room door, I can see this child is ill—not critically so, but still significantly ill. As you read in previous chapters, having an innate sense for when a child is seriously ill is the best test there is for detecting a serious condition. This is a knack that takes time to acquire, but experienced parents are often as apt to have it as are physicians. This mother clearly has the knack, because the first thing she tells me is this: "He's sick and getting sicker by the day."

Her son, she says, has been sick for some time. She is not sure how long, but she first noticed something definite six weeks previously when his clothes did not fit anymore—he had lost weight. She also noticed that his appetite had decreased, he just wanted to nap when he got home from school, and he started to have fevers nearly every night of 101 degrees. She took him to a doctor at a walk-in clinic, who found nothing wrong.

When the boy began to cough, however, she returned with him to the clinic. This time the doctor took an X-ray, even though he did not find anything abnormal on the child's examination other than a weight loss of a pound from his previous visit. The X-ray showed an abnormal white patch, an *infiltrate*, that the doctor interpreted as pneumonia; he prescribed ten days of an oral antibiotic. The medicine seemed to make the child feel better after a couple of days, but he still had a mild fever nearly every day. The cough persisted; it was worse at night and did not bring up any phlegm.

The mother brought her son back to the doctor a third time when the antibiotics had all been taken. The doctor heard her story, took another X-ray, which this time showed a new, but smaller infiltrate in another part of the lung. He prescribed a different antibiotic. That was over a week ago, and although the child is still taking the second antibiotic, he feels no better. His mother thinks he is worse.

The reasons she came to the emergency department were twofold: that morning the child coughed up a couple of tablespoon's worth of bright red blood, and second, the mother was exasperated with the doctor because she did not think he was taking her child's illness seriously enough and was not really listening to her.

I do not know how sick the child looked when he saw the other doctor, of course, but after several weeks of illness the boy is now obviously sick with something. His skin is sallow and his face looks gaunt. His gaze is dull and apathetic as his mother talks to me.

The remainder of the history the mother gives me does not bring anything further of importance to light. The child had always been healthy, and the social history showed no travel or unusual exposures to infections. I do a detailed systems review but turn up nothing else—no abdominal complaints, no headache, no rashes, no painful or swollen joints. These things are what doctors call significant negatives; their absence can be as helpful as discovering they are present.

When I examine the child, I also do not find much more than I already knew—that he is a sick boy with something wrong. The time course of this child's illness is what we call *subacute*, meaning not acute but not really chronic, either. In chapter 4 you read about useful screening laboratory tests, things that can help us narrow our suspicions about what is wrong. Ideal screening tests for disease are *sensitive*, meaning they do not miss much, but they are not necessarily very *specific*, meaning an abnormality found by such a test mostly tells us only to search further for a cause. They also should not be very risky to the child. We do not have a perfect set of screening tests, but the combination of complete blood count, chemistry panel with liver function tests, and urinalysis is a safe and often helpful way to see if something serious is going on. I order these tests on the child, along with a chest X-ray because I already know he has had an abnormality in his lungs.

The test results come back within an hour, and they are all abnormal. Even though his cough is better at the moment and he has no other respiratory symptoms like fast breathing or shortness of breath, his chest X-ray shows patchy areas of infiltrates throughout both his lungs. The picture is indicative of one we might see in a patient with pneumonia, but it also is consistent with other kinds of inflammation in the lungs.

His blood count shows that he is anemic, and the measurement of the size of his red blood cells suggests what we call an anemia of chronic disease, meaning one not caused by insufficient iron in the diet or by excessive bleeding somewhere. His kind of anemia is one we see in people who are just generally ill from any one of a long list of chronic problems; the bone marrow of sick people tends to quit making red blood cells normally. So his blood count does not tell me specifically what he has, but it does confirm that there is something significant wrong.

His blood chemistry panel is also abnormal; it shows evidence of significant problems with his kidneys. His creatinine, a measure of how well the kidneys are filtering body wastes from the blood, is four times what it should be. His other chemistries are also mildly abnormal, reflecting how important the kidneys are at maintaining the chemical balance of our bodies.

Finally, the urinalysis confirms something is very wrong with the boy's kidneys. Normally there are no blood cells in the urine. When the kidneys or bladder become irritated or inflamed, however, we see either white or red blood cells in the urine. If the kidneys are especially inflamed, we see packed deposits of red blood cells called *casts*; these represent oozing of blood from the circulation into the kidney tubes where urine normally forms. The laboratory technician sees many red cell casts in the child's urine when she looks at it under a microscope.

When I see all these abnormal tests, I formulate a differential diagnosis list that can explain them all, trying, as always, to contain everything in a one-disease box. Meanwhile, though, it is clear to me the child is too sick to go home, and the disorders I am considering are all serious ones that will need complicated therapies; I admit this child to the hospital for more tests, meanwhile giving him some intravenous fluids because he has not been drinking well for the past day.

Summarizing what we know, this is a child who has been ill for weeks with fevers, weight loss, and general fatigue and malaise. He has a cough, with at least one episode of coughing up blood, and multiple infiltrates on his chest X-ray that two rounds of antibiotics did nothing to help. He has an anemia of chronic disease and blood chemistry findings that point us to the kidneys. To encompass all this in a diagnosis, we need to come up with a disorder that particularly involves the lungs and the kidneys but also the whole body, and comes on subacutely. We also know this child is seriously ill.

As it turns out, several diseases qualify for the differential diagnosis list. One of a long list of obscure infections could be responsible for this boy's condition. One of these is something called *endocarditis*, an infection of the heart that secondarily affects the whole body. There are other possibilities. The immune system is what protects our body from foreign invaders, such as bacteria. Sometimes, however, for unknown reasons the immune system attacks the person's own body, as you read in chapter eight— rheumatologists are the experts in these autoimmune disorders. This child's problem could very well be caused one of those conditions. But whatever it is, a child like this needs to be admitted to the hospital, where we will have a better chance to figure out what is wrong and treat it appropriately.

We eventually determine that this child has a rare disease called *Wegener's granulomatosis*. Its cause is unknown, but it is one of a family of rare diseases called *vasculitis*, inflammation of the blood vessels. The disease affects the whole body but is particularly prone to involve the lungs and the kidneys, probably because those organs are especially rich in blood vessels. The inflamed vessels bleed, which is why the boy had bleeding into his lungs, and which is reflected by the infiltrates and bloody cough. He also had bleeding into his kidneys, indicated by the red cell casts in his urine. We diagnose these diseases using special blood tests and often a *biopsy*, a sample of involved tissue that we look at under a microscope. Kidney biopsies are relatively easy to do through a needle; lung biopsies are more involved. Patients with vasculitis need the care of subspecialists, who typically use powerful (and sometimes risky) medications to treat them.

We have now moved from a child with a common disease, to an uncommon one, and finally to a distinctly rare disease. A key message of this last case is that even rare diseases usually first manifest themselves with common complaints, sometimes quite vague and ill-defined symptoms. As a parent, the best way to help a doctor evaluate your child is not to search the library or Internet for obscure diseases that might explain your child's symptoms; the best way to help is to observe closely and be particularly systematic in your observations. This is what doctors are trained to do, and you can learn to do it too.

CASE FIVE

Our final case also concerns a boy who has had chronic symptoms, as I find when I scan the nurse's triage note: "Four-year-old boy with periodic mental status changes—happening again today." This is a highly unusual chief complaint. What a physician means by mental status change is an alteration in awareness of one's surroundings. The term describes a continuum ranging from mild confusion all the way to a deep coma. As I read this, I doubt the child is in a coma—those children typically come to the emergency department in an ambulance with lights and sirens—but the story already gets my attention as the most unusual one I have heard yet today.

In the examining room, I find the child dozing, apparently comfortably, on the cot. His mother stands beside him. From the nursing record I already know that the child's vital signs, his temperature, pulse, and most importantly his respiratory pattern and oxygen saturations, are in the normal, safe range. He appears at first glance to be simply drowsy, opening his eyes briefly when he hears me come into the room, then closing them to doze off again.

His mother jumps quickly into the interview, barely giving me a chance to introduce myself: "You see, this is how he gets!" She continues, telling me that her son has had four episodes of becoming excessively drowsy for anywhere from four to twelve hours. He does not complain of any particular discomfort when this happens, such as headache or nausea. She says that the first two of the spells followed close behind viral respiratory infections, but the next one, as well as the current one, came apparently out of the blue; he has not been sick lately in any other way or done anything outside his usual activities.

The first two times it happened, she brought him to the doctor, and on both occasions she was told that the child's mild disorientation was from the viral illness and would pass quickly, which it did both times. The third time, the child had just seemed groggy one morning but was better by evening; she did not take him to the doctor because there were no other symptoms and the spell passed.

This morning, however, she found her son nearly unresponsive in his bed when she went into his room to discover why he was not up and playing, as he usually was by that time. When she awakened him by shaking his shoulder, he at first did not seem to recognize her, but then he told her he wanted to sleep some more. He did not complain of anything when she asked him if anything hurt. She got him out of bed, and although he could stand, he seemed a little unsteady on his feet. She then brought him to the emergency department, where he has continued to be drowsy, although she thinks he may be a little better by this time.

Before I hear anything else, I am formulating a working differential diagnosis list in my mind, and for all the items on it, additional history is key. A story like this is consistent with intoxication or poisoning from something that affects the brain, although several of these episodes spanning a period of time make that diagnosis less likely. If there were a single instance, ingestion of something that alters awareness would be at the top of my list. I ask the mother about this, and also if anyone in the household is taking any medicines the boy could have gotten into. The mother takes a thyroid medicine, the boy's father a medicine for blood pressure, and his older brother takes medicine for hyperactivity.

This information catches my attention. Although antihyperactivity medicines generally make a normal child overstimulated, not somnolent, there are several blood pressure medicines that can make children lethargic. The mother does not know what the medicine is, but she will check with her husband, who will see if all the pills are accounted for. Even so, both the mother and I doubt that this the reason, since the child was well when he went to bed and the mother is certain she would have heard him get out of bed during the night. Besides, all the pills—both the blood pressure medicine and the hyperactivity medicine—are kept in the parents' bathroom, not the child's.

I also have on my evolving list some kind of seizure, because there are unusual varieties that manifest themselves by altering a child's awareness. This seems unlikely, though, because those kinds of seizures are generally quite brief, lasting only seconds to a minute. Seizures can affect awareness for several hours after they are over, but those kinds of seizures are quite obvious when they are happening, so that also makes the possibility unlikely. Still, I keep it on my list along with the possibility of an ingestion of a toxic substance.

I then turn to the family history, social history, and systems review. The mother tells me the boy has a first cousin, the son of her sister, who has some ill-defined kind of neurological problem; the child lives far away, however, and the mother does not know any more than that. The family lives in the city in a newer house, so this child would not seem to have any opportunity for exposure to things like lead paint (which affects the brain) or toxic farm chemicals. His systems review shows him to be generally normal, although the mother says that his preschool teacher recently told her she was concerned that the boy was behind the other children in his learning skills. The teacher suggested an evaluation by a pediatrician, although the mother had not done that yet.

I next examine the child. His mental status is about what it had been for the previous couple of hours; he opens his eyes when I talk to him and complains if I poke him or pinch him, but he will not answer questions. I ask him if he knows where he is and who is with him; he does not recognize the room as being in the hospital, but he does recognize his mother. The rest of the boy's physical examination is completely normal.

Summarizing, we have a generally healthy boy who has experienced several discrete, well-observed spells of altered mental state. Two of these were associated with viral infections, but two of them were not. He has the potential for exposure to at least one medication that could cause similar symptoms, but it is difficult to see how this could have happened, and the rest of his daily environment does not contain anything toxic. There is a possibility that the boy's overall development is not entirely normal, and he has a male cousin who has some kind of neurological problem. His physical examination is unhelpful in deciding what this is. The history, however, tells me what I need to find this out in order to proceed logically to diagnose the problem.

The history makes me highly suspicious that this child has one of several inherited disorders that affect how the body processes protein, the building blocks of the body's cells. These are called *urea cycle disorders*, named after the urea cycle, the metabolic pathway that breaks down proteins. There are other rare metabolic diseases that could cause these symptoms, all of which together we call *inborn errors of metabolism*. I do, of course, also remember the dictum that something strange is more likely to be an uncommon manifestation of a common thing than a rare thing. In this case the common thing would be a drug or toxin ingestion, so I perform the appropriate tests for that possibility. But I also test for rare diseases.

The most useful screening test for a urea cycle problem is a blood ammonia level, so I order that. Ammonia is a direct suppressant of brain function, which usually makes children progressively sleepy, until they are in an actual coma if the level gets high enough. There are also several other blood and urine tests that will help me determine if the boy has any other kind of inborn error. These tests are most useful when the child is actually having symptoms, so now is a good time to get them done. The blood ammonia test and blood sugar levels are the only ones that come back quickly (many of the others take days), and they are the most important practical ones anyway; his ammonia is far too high. My next move is to arrange to admit the child to the hospital and to call for help from one of my subspecialty colleagues, in this case a pediatric endocrinologist.

This child does indeed turn out to have an inherited problem with his urea cycle metabolic pathway; he has *ornithine transcarbamylase deficiency*, named for one of the enzymes in the cycle. Poor function of the enzyme makes ammonia build up in the body.

Some children have severe problems, others less severe, depending upon how deficient their enzyme is. Spells of worsening symptoms can happen spontaneously, but body stress, such as with an acute infection, is a common trigger. A chronically high ammonia level is hard on the nervous system, so many children have some degree of developmental delay.

This last case is a real zebra, but every doctor knows that sometimes hoofbeats really do come from zebras, so we always need to be listening for them, at least in the back of our minds. This case is an excellent example of how all aspects of the history—the present, past, family, social, and systems review—come together to guide what we do. It was the combination of all these things that made me suspect the diagnosis.

All of these cases show you, through a doctor's eyes, how our evaluation of your child begins even before we have seen him. As soon as we lay eyes on you and your child, we begin to gather information, even before we have said anything and certainly before we begin our examination. In these days when both parents and doctors are more and more pressed for time, you as a parent can have a substantial, even crucial effect on your child's medical evaluation. You can do this by seeing the situation as a doctor sees it and then communicating as doctors communicate. Now you know how, and I encourage you to practice your newfound skills. Your child will benefit and your doctor will thank you.

INDEX

osteopathic, 183
proprietary, 179
requirements, 184
scrotum, 82
sedatives, 114, 118, 121
seizure, 119, 143, 164, 223
sepsis, 96
Septra, 162
Shaw, George Bernard, 191
sign
  peritoneal, 81
  physical, 40
  vital, 66
Singulair, 168
sinusitis, 74
skin, 83, 141–42
  testing, 170
skull, 69, 98
social history (SH), 48–49, 54
sodium, 94
sonar, 114
sore throat, 74, 129
specialists. *See* subspecialists
spinal cord, 98
spinal tap, 98
spleen, 79, 81, 87
steroids, 18, 165, 167, 175
  inhaled, 167
  nasal, 170
  oral, 21, 53
stethoscope, 62, 66, 77, 78, 131
stimulants for ADHD, 174
stomach, 79, 136
stomatitis

aphthous, 130
herpes, 129
strep throat, 74, 129, 268–72
Streptococcus pyogenes, 74
stridor, 18
subacute, definition of, 280
subspecialists, 124, 208, 230–35
Sudafed, 170
Sulamyd, 162
sulfonamide, 162
superior, *cephalad*, 38
Suprax, 161
surgeon, 62, 135
  ear, nose, and throat (ENT), 228
  orthopedic, 226
  pediatric, 225
  urological, 227
surgical abdomen, 136
symptom, 40
syringe, 95
system
  cardiovascular, 51
  constitutional, 51
  ears, nose, and throat (ENT), 51
  endocrine, 52
  gastrointestinal, 52
  genitourinary, 52
  hematological, 52
  musculoskeletal, 52
  neurological, 52
  ocular, 51
  respiratory, 52
  skin, 52
systole, 66

vomiting, 23, 133
  color and consistency of coffee
    grounds, 136

weakness, 143
Wegener's granulomatosis,
  278–83
wheezing, 18, 53, 77, 131, 166,
  169
whooping cough, 162
windpipe, 22

worms, 105

x-ray, 171. *See also* tests, x-ray
  figure of, 107
  safety of, 109

Zantac, 172
Zion, Libby, 186
Zovirax, 163
Zyrtec, 169